Recent Advances in Alzheimer Research

(*Volume 3*)

Alzheimer Disease: Pathological and Clinical Findings

Edited by

Blas Gil-Extremera

Department of Medicine, Universidad de Granada, Granada, Spain

Recent Advances in Alzheimer Research

Volume # 3

Alzheimer Disease: Pathological and Clinical Findings

Editor: Blas Gil-Extremera

ISSN (Online): 2452-2562

ISSN (Print): 2452-2554

ISBN (Online): 978-981-14-0513-6

ISBN (Print): 978-981-14-0512-9

need for a court order if at any point you breach any terms of this License Agreement. In no event will any delay or failure by Bentham Science Publishers in enforcing your compliance with this License Agreement constitute a waiver of any of its rights.

3. You acknowledge that you have read this License Agreement, and agree to be bound by its terms and conditions. To the extent that any other terms and conditions presented on any website of Bentham Science Publishers conflict with, or are inconsistent with, the terms and conditions set out in this License Agreement, you acknowledge that the terms and conditions set out in this License Agreement shall prevail.

Bentham Science Publishers Pte. Ltd.
80 Robinson Road #02-00
Singapore 068898
Singapore
Email: subscriptions@benthamscience.net

BENTHAM SCIENCE

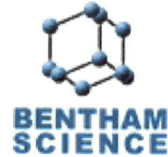

CONTENTS

PREFACE

Alzheimer's disease was named after Dr. Alois Alzheimer (1864-1915) in 1906 who described two important microscopic findings: neuritic plaques and neurofibrillary tangles in the brain of a 55-year old female, who died from dementia. These two lesions are characteristic but not pathognomonic of the disease. Alzheimer's disease is the most common form of dementia in the Western countries. The origin of the disease is still unclear although it has been demonstrated that ageing in the major risk factor. The management of this neurologic disorder is frustrating since, until now, no specific and curative treatment has been found, and so far, the only possibility to fight against the disease is to try to improve as much as possible the symptoms and the neurologic effects of the disease.

Bentham e-Book Editorial had the courtesy to offer to our research group, the invitation to write and update of the Alzheimer's disease. Nine specialized neurologists and general physicians whose expertise are based on dementia and old people diseases have participated in this interesting and exciting project.

This book has nine chapters covering different aspects of the disease such as amyloid hypothesis, symptoms, pain, dysphagia, neuroimaging, brain connectivity, treatment, nutrition and palliative care. I believe that this book can be of great interest for students, physicians, internists, and even for patients, and their families.

Finally, I would like to thank all the authors in this book, also Esperanza Velasco Rodríguez for the preparation of the manuscripts, and the Bentham Publishing Editorial that gave us this valuable opportunity.

Blas Gil-Extremera
Department of Medicine,
Universidad de Granada,
Granada,
Spain

List of Contributors

Andrea R. Vasconcelos	Pharmacology Department, Institute of Biomedical Sciences, University of São Paulo, São Paulo, Brazil
Cristoforo Scavone	Pharmacology Department, Institute of Biomedical Sciences, University of São Paulo, São Paulo, Brazil
Daniel C. Carrettiero	Center of Natural and Human Sciences, Federal University of ABC (UFABC), São Bernardo do Campo, São Paulo, Brazil
Daniel M. Silva	Center for Mathematics, Computation and Cognition, Federal University of ABC (UFABC), São Bernardo do Campo, São Paulo, Brazil
Daniela R. de Oliveira	Center for Mathematics, Computation and Cognition, Federal University of ABC (UFABC), São Bernardo do Campo, São Paulo, Brazil
Elisa M. Kawamoto	Pharmacology Department, Institute of Biomedical Sciences, University of São Paulo, São Paulo, Brazil
Fernanda L. Ribeiro	Center for Mathematics, Computation and Cognition, Federal University of ABC (UFABC), São Bernardo do Campo, São Paulo, Brazil
Fernando A. Oliveira	Center for Mathematics, Computation and Cognition, Federal University of ABC (UFABC), São Bernardo do Campo, São Paulo, Brazil
João C. dos Santos Silva	Center for Mathematics, Computation and Cognition, Federal University of ABC (UFABC), São Bernardo do Campo, São Paulo, Brazil
Laíz C. Silva-Gonçalves	Department of Biophysics, Federal University of São Paulo, São Paulo, Brazil
Luisa Ribeiro-Silva	Department of Biophysics, Federal University of São Paulo, São Paulo, Brazil
Manoel Arcisio-Miranda	Department of Biophysics, Federal University of São Paulo, São Paulo, Brazil
Marcela B. Echeverry	Center for Mathematics, Computation and Cognition, Federal University of ABC (UFABC), São Bernardo do Campo, São Paulo, Brazil
Maria C. Almeida	Center of Natural and Human Sciences, Federal University of ABC (UFABC), São Bernardo do Campo, São Paulo, Brazil
Merari F. R. Ferrari	Department of Genetics and Evolutionary Biology, Institute for Biosciences, University of Sao Paulo, Sao Paulo, Brazil
Paula F. Kinoshita	Pharmacology Department, Institute of Biomedical Sciences, University of São Paulo, São Paulo, Brazil
Rolf M. Paninka	Department of Biophysics, Federal University of São Paulo, São Paulo, Brazil
Samanta Rodrigues	Center for Mathematics, Computation and Cognition, Federal University of ABC (UFABC), São Bernardo do Campo, São Paulo, Brazil
Sonia G. Prieto	Center for Mathematics, Computation and Cognition, Federal University of ABC (UFABC), São Bernardo do Campo, São Paulo, Brazil
Tatiana L. Ferreira	Center for Mathematics, Computation and Cognition, Federal University of ABC (UFABC), São Bernardo do Campo, São Paulo, Brazil
Vitor S. Alves	Center for Mathematics, Computation and Cognition, Federal University of ABC (UFABC), São Bernardo do Campo, São Paulo, Brazil

CHAPTER 1

Amyloid Hypothesis in Alzheimer´s Disease

Maria Sagrario Manzano Palomo[*]

Neurology Department, Infanta Leonor Hospital, Madrid, Spain

Abstract: Alzheimer's disease (AD) is a neurodegenerative condition which is highly prevalent. According to the World Health Organization (WHO) estimates, the overall projected prevalence in worldwide will reach 132 million patients by 2050. Amyloid hypothesis described in 90´s by Hardy et al, is the main therapeutic target. Since acetylcholinesterase inhibitors as symptomatic treatment, drug development for AD has been disappointing. All drugs in completed phase 2 and phase 3 trials have failed.

So, the question is, what´s wrong about this hypothesis and the immunotherapy approach? These compounds aimed at reducing Aβ formation and plaques do not restore cognition although removes amyloid plaques in PET amyloid scans.

This paper tries to discuss all the aspects and describe the current situation and the future goals.

Keywords: Amyloid-β, Alzheimer's Disease, Immunotherapy, New Therapies, Tau Protein.

INTRODUCTION

Alzheimer's disease (AD) is a neurodegenerative condition which is highly prevalent in old age [1 - 4]. Costs for care of older people will continue to increase and that the number of diagnosed dementia and will reach 132 million patients according to The World Health Organization (WHO) and Alzheimer Disease International (ADI) [2, 3]. According to the Alzheimer's Association, 13% of people over 65 suffer from this disease in developed countries, and is increasing in developing countries. This condition has a great socio-economic impact, and this would also clearly lead to increased economic burden to healthcare systems all over the world [1 - 4].

AD has an insidious onset focused on episodic memory lost. Cognitive symptoms appear late in progression of the disease so it´s quite difficult achieve effective

[*] **Corresponding author Maria Sagrario Manzano Palomo:** Neurology Department, Infanta Cristina Hospital, Madrid, Spain; Tel: +629124822; E-mail: sagmanpal@gmail.com

Blas Gil-Extremera (Ed.)

therapies. The preclinical phase of the disease includes more than one or two decades of changes in the brain without any king of symptomatology. At the diagnostic stage, there is already extensive deposition of Aβ, neurofibrillary tangles, synaptic lost and cell death, each of which might contribute to the main neuropsychological hallmark, episodic memory loss [5].

Aging as a trigger of proteinopathies, is the principal risk factor for sporadic AD. Other well known risk factors include depression in midlife, low education level, obesity, hypertension in the midlife, dyslipidemia, metabolic syndrome and diabetes have also been identified [5 - 8].

Aging brain is more vulnerable to downstream insults due to another reason or could be a reason that compromises clearance mechanism, predisposing to the proteinopathy [9].

The treatment strategies are focused on hypotheses aimed at explaining the origins of AD. There are many hypothesis, first of all being amyloid cascade.

The hypotheses are:

  a. amyloid cascade hypothesis,
  b. cholinergic hypothesis,
  c. dendritic hypothesis,
  d. mitochondrial cascade hypothesis,
  e. metabolic hypothesis,
  f. oxidative stress,
  g. neuro inflammation,
  h. synapsis dysfunction,
  i. others

Immunotherapies are separated into passive and active vaccine approaches. In an active vaccine approach, a pathogenic agent is injected into the patient. That provokes a response in the innate immune system. In a passive one, a specific antibody against the antigen is injected trying to remove antibody-bound ligand.

In this review, the main goal is trying to focus on amyloid hypothesis, because the principal targets and clinical trials of the compounds (passive vaccine approach) aimed at reducing Aβ formation and plaques.

The amyloid hypothesis has the key of the pathogenesis of AD, and has guided efforts to find effective treatments.

We make some comments about tau protein target because the future in therapeutics focused on AD would pass to considered combination strategies.

AMYLOID AS THERAPEUTIC TARGET IN AD

Aβ peptide is derived from proteolysis of APP (*amyloid precursor protein*). It's an integral transmembrane protein and it's found in different cell types (neurons, glial cells) [9]. APP is processed *via* cleavage by secretases, α, β, and γ secretase enzyme protein complexes, into smaller peptide fragments, one of which is Aβ.

A pathological hallmark of AD brain pathology is the accumulation of small spherical structures called amyloid plaques or senile plaques (SP). These plaques are composed of insoluble fibrils formed by the protein fragment Aβ. (The toxic spicy considered is Aβ42).

AMYLOID CASCADE HYPOTHESIS: A BRIEF REVIEW

The 'amyloid cascade hypothesis' (ACH) [10] is the pathological model of AD with more influence in the last 25 years. See Fig. (**1**).

The original formulation of the hypothesis was the result of the discovery of Aβ.

Aβ is the most important constituent of senile plaques (SP). The mutations of the amyloid precursor protein (APP) gene is associated to early-onset familial AD (FAD) [10]. There have been many opinions, difficult to reconcile among researches since its publication. One of them, is elated to transgenic mice. In these animal models, genes overexpress amyloid precursor protein (APP), and do not reproduce the cascade as it's known [11]. Another one, is that Aβ and tau could be the final consequence of neurodegeneration (oxidative stress) more than its cause. And another observation is, for example, that in late-onset AD, the central pathological role for Aβ is not clear in many studies using biomarkers of neuronal injury. These considerations suggest a more complex relationship between Aβ, tau, and AD pathogenesis.

The original formulation of the ACH was proposed by Hardy and Higgins [10], see Fig. (**1**). These are, in a brief version, many observations resulted in the formulation and development of the hypothesis, and causes of its interpretation and limitations [11]. We sum up them in order to a better understanding of it:

1. Aβ was is the most important molecular constituent of SP.
2. In the first stages, the proteolytic processing of APP is altered at last it's accumulated.
3. Early-onset FAD are associated to APP gene mutations.

4. APP processing produces Aβ peptides.
   a. cleavage by βACE1.
   b. cleavage by γ-secretase.
      Aβ soluble oligomers are toxic. They could vary with a type of mutant. It provides a genetic basis for variations in pathogenesis observed among FAD cases.
5. The most common form of early-onset FAD is due to presenilin (PSEN) genes, PSEN1 and PSEN2 mutations.
6. Down's syndrome (DS) replicates "*in vivo*" many of the features of AD pathology.
7. Some of Aβ peptides are toxic. They could induce cell death, depending on cell type.
8. Aβ may induce the phosphorylation of tau.
9. Senile plaques and NFT could acquire those known 'secondary' constituents. They may be involved in the maturation of Aβ deposits and formation of SP.

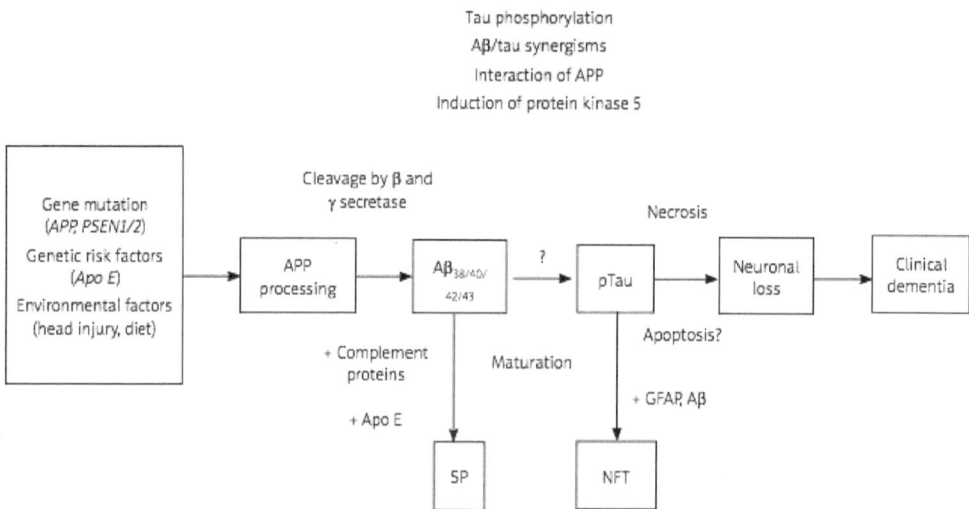

Tau phosphorylation
Aβ/tau synergisms
Interaction of APP
Induction of protein kinase 5

Aβ – β-amyloid, Apo E – apolipoprotein E, APP – amyloid precursor protein, GFAP – glial fibrillary acidic protein, PSEN1/2 – presenilin genes 1 and 2, NFT – neurofibrillary tangles, pTau – hyperphosphorylated tau, SP – senile plaques

Fig. (1). Amyloid Cascade Hypothesis [11].

AMYLOID AS THERAPEUTIC TARGET

The majority of clinical trials with target Aβ drugs have not reached the primary endpoints and have, in some cases, serious side-effects. Removed amyloid does not restore cognition.

There is not a direct correlation between amyloid plaque burden and memory loss in AD. It demonstrates that neurotoxicity not only depends on the insoluble Aβ oligomers [12 - 14], but also depends on the soluble oligomers and insoluble fibrils Aβ.

Thus, the question about Aβ (production or clearance) and if it could be a good target for treatment, is still unknown. Efforts focused in translational research are essential.

It is believed that Aβ is generated in a continuous way and its aggregation and plaque deposition depends on its concentration. Excessive accumulation of both soluble oligomers and insoluble fibrils Aβ could be the result of aberrant APP processing by *β*- and *γ*-secretase enzymes. It could be produces by an inefficient removal of toxic Aβ species newly generated [15 - 22].

A more comprehensive would be to compare AD with coronary disease. Beyond being a proteinopathy, AD disrupts a networking of the whole brain. In this way, atherosclerotic heart disease is as an excellent example of another human disease caused by long-term accumulation of a metabolite: cholesterol. Cholesterol accumulation in coronary arteries occurs decades before the first symptoms, the same that amyloid in the brain. If a good treatment for hypercholesterolemia is started early during the process, the impact of on atherosclerotic heart disease could be so healthy as many studies have published; however, lowering cholesterol after a heart failure has minimal benefit in this kind of patient, as secondary prevention strategy [23, 25].

Similarly, the amyloid hypothesis and the benefit in symptomatic AD preventing its accumulation could be the solution. By inference, if the only therapeutic target is Aβ accumulation, it could show less efficacy during the course of the disease and the underlying pathology progresses [24, 26]. This hypothesis is widely explained in the review of Golde [25].

REMOVE AMYLOID-B HAVE NOT YET RESTORE COGNITION

Current Active Anti-b-Amyloid Immunotherapy for Alzheimer's Disease

Aβ peptide contributes to the cause and progression of AD, and is one of the main therapeutic target of this complex disease. Elevated levels of Aβ probably underlie its pathogenicity, so the strategies are focused on: the aberrant generation of Aβ and the clearance mechanisms [25].

The active or passive vaccination stimulates Ab clearance from the AD brain and represents the most innovative approach of anti-Alzheimer's disease therapy [26 - 28].

The first Phase IIa clinical trial for an active AD vaccine, AN1792, was performed in 2002 (*ELAN, Dublin, Ireland, and Wyeth, PA, USA*). It contained the full-length Aβ42 peptide. It demonstrated some beneficial effects, but some patients developed meningoencephalitis (6% of the treated group) [26, 27], so the clinical trial was failure.

The failure of AN1792, CAD106 ten years after, carried out the second generation of active Ab immunotherapy [29].

Another two active immunizations, ACC-001 (vanutide cridificar) and Affitope AD02 [30] are currently in Phase II clinical trials. Early clinical data from Phase I trials confirmed positive antibody responses with no adverse autoimmune inflammation signs (see Table **1**).

Table 1. Active immunotherapy in AD. Modify www.alzforum.org.

Name	Synonyms	FDA Status	Company	Target Type	Therapy Type	Condition	Approved For
ACI-24	Pal1-15 acetate salt	1/2, 1	AC Immune SA	Amyloid-Related	Immunotherapy (active)	Alzheimer's Disease, Down's Syndrome	
AN-1792	AIP 001	Discontinued	Janssen, Pfizer	Amyloid-Related	Immunotherapy (active)	Alzheimer's Disease	None
Affitope AD02		2	AFFiRiS AG	Amyloid-Related	Immunotherapy (active)	Alzheimer's Disease	
CAD106		2/3	Novartis Pharmaceuticals Corporation	Amyloid-Related	Immunotherapy (active)	Alzheimer's Disease	None
Vanutide cridificar	ACC-001, PF-05236806	Discontinued	Janssen	Amyloid-Related	Immunotherapy (active)	Alzheimer's Disease	None

Further Phase II trials are needed for these active immunization therapies [30].

Current Passive Anti-b-Amyloid Immunotherapy for Alzheimer's Disease

Passive immunization is focused on introducing manufactured humanized antibodies into the patients.

Bapineuzumab (AAB-001) represents the more characteristic of them. It is a fully humanized monoclonal antibody directed against the N-terminus of Aß, recognizing the Ab1–5 regions [31]. No significant clinical benefits have been reported in two large Phase III clinical trials, leading to the discontinuation of all Phase III clinical trials.

Other are solanezumab (*Eli Lilly and Co., IN, USA and Hoffmann-LaRoche, Basel, Switzerland*) gantenerumab (*Hoffmann-LaRoche*), crenezumab (*Genentech, CA, USA*), and aducanumab (*Biogen Idec, MA, USA*), CAD106 (*Novartis; NCT02565511*) and ACC-001 (*Janssen, Pfizer; NCT01284387*) [30]. Among these, solanezumab was failure in December 2016 [28], and it is ongoing in A4 trial and DIAN project (see Table **2**).

Thus, there has been no definitive results about targeting Aβ in symptomatic AD will have symptomatic benefit.

Aducanumab (Biogen Idec, MA, USA) is the first antibody with the property of being highly selective of Aβ aggregate (soluble oligomers and insoluble fibrils, but not monomers) and, in the reported Phase 1b study, shows clear evidence for reducing amyloid burden in amyloid PET scans and it could have some cognitive and functional benefit [32, 33]. The aducanumab phase 3 study will have outcomes in one or two years.

Secretase inhibitors also have been tested. The enzyme γ-secretase was regarded as a valid therapeutic target trying to inhibit its activity, (avagacestat and semagacestat) failed. The causes were a high degree of toxicity (notch-signaling damage), and worsening of cognition [34].

β-secretase, including the form known as BACE1, cleaves APP extracellularly to produce Aβ peptides. The development of BACE1 inhibitors drugs is carrying out in trials in patient with prodromal AD or AD dementia, or indeed in preclinical stages. The most advanced is verubecestat (*MK-8931; Merck*), which is in combination phase 2/3 trials for either prodromal AD or mild-to-moderate AD dementia. It has been reported failure outcome in early AD dementia. Outcomes are expected in this year [35].

Table 2. Passive immunotherapy in AD. Modify www.alzforum.org.

Name	Synonyms	FDA Status	Company	Target Type	Therapy Type	Condition	Approved for
AAB-003	PF-05236812	1	Janssen, Pfizer	Amyloid-Related	Immunotherapy (passive)	Alzheimer's Disease	
Aducanumab	BIIB037	3	Biogen	Amyloid-Related	Immunotherapy (passive)	Alzheimer's Disease	
BAN2401		2	Biogen, Eisai Co., Ltd.	Amyloid-Related	Immunotherapy (passive)	Alzheimer's Disease	
Bapineuzumab	AAB-001	Discontinued	Janssen, Pfizer	Amyloid-Related	Immunotherapy (passive)	Alzheimer's Disease	
Crenezumab	MABT5102A, RG7412	3	Genentech	Amyloid-Related	Immunotherapy (passive)	Alzheimer's Disease	None
GSK933776		Inactive	GlaxoSmithKline (GSK)	Amyloid-Related	Immunotherapy (passive)	Alzheimer's Disease	

(Table 2) cont.....

Name	Synonyms	FDA Status	Company	Target Type	Therapy Type	Condition	Approved for
Gammagard®	Intravenous Immunoglobulin, IVIg	Discontinued	Baxter Healthcare	Amyloid-Related, Inflammation	Immunotherapy (passive)	Alzheimer's Disease	Immunodeficiency conditions
Gamunex	Intravenous Immunoglobulin, Human Albumin Combined With Flebogamma	2/3	Grifols Biologicals Inc.	Amyloid-Related, Inflammation	Immunotherapy (passive)	Alzheimer's Disease	Immunodeficiency, chronic inflammatory demyelinating neuropathy
Gantenerumab	RO4909832, RG1450	3	Chugai Pharmaceutical Co., Ltd., Hoffmann-La Roche	Amyloid-Related	Immunotherapy (passive)	Alzheimer's Disease	
LY3002813	N3pG-Aβ Monoclonal Antibody	1	Eli Lilly & Co.	Amyloid-Related	Immunotherapy (passive)	Alzheimer's Disease	
MEDI1814		1	AstraZeneca	Amyloid-Related	Immunotherapy (passive)	Alzheimer's Disease	
Octagam®10%	Intravenous Immunoglobulin, NewGam	Inactive, Inactive	Octapharma	Amyloid-Related, Inflammation	Immunotherapy (passive)	Alzheimer's Disease, Mild Cognitive Impairment	Immunodeficiency disorders
Ponezumab	PF-04360365	Discontinued, 2	Pfizer	Amyloid-Related	Immunotherapy (passive)	Alzheimer's Disease, Cerebral Amyloid Angiopathy	None
SAR228810		1	Sanofi	Amyloid-Related	Immunotherapy (passive)	Alzheimer's Disease	
Solanezumab	LY2062430	3	Eli Lilly & Co.	Amyloid-Related	Immunotherapy (passive)	Alzheimer's Disease	None

TAU-BASED TREATMENTS

Tau is an intracellular protein to assist in stability of the cytoarchitecture, especially in neurons. It binds to microtubules to provide structural support for axons, and it also facilitates trafficking of important intracellular compounds and organelles.

Tau and its hyperphosphorylated version are the main constituent of intracellular neurofibrillary tangles, one of the main hallmark of AD. Tau pathology in AD spreads from the entorhinal cortex, followed by hippocampal and cortical areas [36]. The specific stage of tau pathology also correlates well with cognitive abilities [37, 38].

Nowadays, it is considered a main player in this disease and others, for example, frontotemporal dementia, and all the efforts have focused on developing inhibitors of the enzymes tau kinases, which phosphorylate the protein and so on, would probably reach to the therapeutic target in neurodegenerative diseases *via* combination strategies [39].

The main topic of this review is Aβ. But it's necessary to talk about tau, because the combination strategies could be, the future in AD therapeutics.

The pathogenic link between Aβ deposition and tau pathology—and their contributions to neurodegeneration, remain unclear.

Drugs that reduce hyperphosphorylation of tau protein, or the fibrillation or deposition of tau, are in development. These effects have been shown *in vitro* for several drugs.

Rember was the first anti-tau oral drug that reached to phase III but, it was not efficacious (see www.alzforum.org).

Another new formulation of methylene blue, TRx0237 (LMTX; TauRx Therapeutics), is being tested in a phase 3 trial of 833 patients with mild-to-moderate AD, with patients followed up for 12 months (NCT01689246), and a phase 2 trial of 500 patients with mild frontotemporal dementia, followed up for 18 months (*NCT01626378*). Outcomes of both trials are expected in this year (see Table **3**).

Table 3. Therapeutics related to tau. Modified www.alzforum.org.

Name	Synonyms	FDA Status	Company	Target Type	Therapy Type	Condition	Approved For
AADvac-1	Axon peptide 108 conjugated to KLH	1	Axon Neuroscience SE	Tau	Immunotherapy (active)	Alzheimer's Disease	
ACI-35		1	AC Immune SA, Janssen	Tau	Immunotherapy (active)	Alzheimer's Disease	
BMS-986168	IPN007	1	Bristol-Myers Squibb	Tau	Immunotherapy (passive)	Progressive Supranuclear Palsy	
C2N 8E12	ABBV-8E12	1	AbbVie, C2N Diagnostics, LLC	Tau	Immunotherapy (passive)	Progressive Supranuclear Palsy	
Rember TM	Methylene Blue, methylthioninium (MT), TRx-0014, Tau aggregation inhibitor (TAI)	Discontinued	TauRx Therapeutics Ltd	Tau	Small Molecule	Alzheimer's Disease	Methylene Blue predates FDA. Used for treatment of malaria and methemoglobinemia.

(Table 3) cont.....

Name	Synonyms	FDA Status	Company	Target Type	Therapy Type	Condition	Approved For
TPI 287		1, 1, 1	Cortice Biosciences	Tau	Small Molecule	Alzheimer's Disease, Corticobasal Degeneration, Progressive Supranuclear Palsy	
TRx0237	LMT-X, LMTM, Methylene Blue, Tau aggregation inhibitor (TAI)	3, 3	TauRx Therapeutics Ltd	Tau	Small Molecule	Alzheimer's Disease, Frontotemporal Dementia	Methylene Blue predates FDA. Used for treatment of malaria and methemoglobinemia.
Tideglusib	NP031112, Nypta®, Zentylor™, Glycogen synthase kinase 3 inhibitor, NP12	Discontinued, Discontinued	Zeltia Group	Tau	Small Molecule	Alzheimer's Disease, Progressive Supranuclear Palsy	

ALZHEIMER´S DISEASE: THE WAY FORWARD IN THERAPEUTIC DEVELOPMENT

We should take into accounts many aspects. Not only research considerations, but also socio-economic and bioethical implications.

This approach about new drugs in AD focused on immunotherapies, raises important questions about the future of drug development for AD, including ethics, costs, biomarkers, social aspects, and long clinical trials participation for people with AD and their families.

New trial designs are needed, but we need improve both basic and translational research.

Biomarkers will be crucial for diagnosis, but nowadays have yet to be validated. We need high levels of sensitivity and specificity, to be clinically useful and also be cost-effectiveness. The risk of false-positive and false-negative cases is present [40]. Challenges in peripheral biomarker (blood biomarkers), are a reality and they will reach in next future. It´s essential in the development of new drugs [25].

Indeed, the high necessity of resources and costs during the predementia period (preclinical and prodromal stages) need to be change for a cost-effectiveness assessment. Another question is if therapy needs to be continuous for the whole life of the patient or require only a few doses, making the therapy more practical to deliver widely (like other vaccines). Financial considerations, even in wealthy countries need to be taken into account as the cost of dementia predicted to be 2 billion dollars by 2050 [25].

Population ageing is a reality and it's occurring worldwide. The multifactorial etiology of dementia in old individuals, including concurrent vascular dementia and different types of neurodegenerative lesions, is a problem to solve in new developing drugs in dementia field. Physical and psychiatric comorbidities are also frequent in advanced age, accompanied by poly-pharmacotherapy (non-optimum use of drugs). It causes anticholinergic and sedative effects in geriatric patients with AD [41, 42].

AD is a 'brain organ failure', and to develop effective therapies for symptomatic AD, we may need to develop a combination approach from the start [24]. Future combination therapies, include multiple therapies trying to restore proteostasis, providing trophic support, restoring neural pathways, providing cognitive enhancement or some combination of these approaches.

A comprehensive and multidisciplinary assessment to every elderly patient is crucial. It's important to enhance the concept of "healthy aging" [43].

FUTURE GOALS

The causes of AD are not well known despite impressive efforts in the past three decades.

Furthermore, the assumption that genetic forms of AD are the same that sporadic ones is a mistake. Late onset AD is an entity different in which concur several injuries difficult to treat with a unique therapeutic approach.

Non-European initiatives such as the API [44] (see www.alzforum.org) study (of one kindred carrying a mutation in *PSEN1*), and the DIAN study [44] (see www.alzforum.org) (of individuals with mutations in *APP*, *PSEN1*, or *PSEN2*) will determine, in the near future, whether clearance of Aβ from the brain is effective in the treatment of familial AD.

For most sporadic, late-onset AD cases, amyloid accumulation is probably a later event that results from other metabolic disruptions. We have information on different pathways that contribute to the disease. A priority for the future is combine strategies, for example anti tau anti-AB drugs.

The identification of patients, that is, not only an AD entity but also AD patients is the first step. Those with similarities could be included in more effective and personalized treatments. Intensification of basic research (translational research) will also result in the identification of new future and realistic goals [45].

CONSENT FOR PUBLICATION

Not applicable.

ACKNOWLEDGEMENTS

Declare none.

CONFLICT OF INTEREST

The author confirms that this chapter contents have no conflict of interest.

REFERENCES

[1]   Santana I, Farinha F, Freitas S, Rodrigues V, Carvalho A. The epidemiology of dementia and Alzheimer disease in Portugal: estimations of prevalence and treatment-costs. Acta Medica Portuguesa 2015; 28(2): 182-8. Neural Plasticity 11.

[2]   Alzheimer's Association Report, "Alzheimer's disease facts and figures Alzheimer's Association. Alzheimers Dement 2015; 11: 332-84.
[PMID: 25984581]

[3]   Prince M, Albanese E, Guerchet M, Prina M. ADI: World Alzheimer Report 2014, Dementia and Risk Reduction: An Analysis of Protective and Modifiable Factors. ADI publisher 2014.

[4]   Chiang K, Koo EH. Emerging therapeutics for Alzheimer's disease. Annu Rev Pharmacol Toxicol 2014; 54: 381-405.
[http://dx.doi.org/10.1146/annurev-pharmtox-011613-135932] [PMID: 24392696]

[5]   Hyman BT, Phelps CH, Beach TG, *et al*. National Institute on Aging-Alzheimer's Association guidelines for the neuropathologic assessment of Alzheimer's disease. Alzheimers Dement 2012; 8(1): 1-13.
[http://dx.doi.org/10.1016/j.jalz.2011.10.007] [PMID: 22265587]

[6]   Castello MA, Soriano S. Rational heterodoxy: cholesterol reformation of the amyloid doctrine. Ageing Res Rev 2013; 12(1): 282-8.
[http://dx.doi.org/10.1016/j.arr.2012.06.007] [PMID: 22771381]

[7]   Castello MA, Soriano S. On the origin of Alzheimer's disease. Trials and tribulations of the amyloid hypothesis. Ageing Res Rev 2014; 13(1): 10-2.
[http://dx.doi.org/10.1016/j.arr.2013.10.001] [PMID: 24252390]

[8]   Drachman DA. The amyloid hypothesis, time to move on: Amyloid is the downstream result, not cause, of Alzheimer's disease. Alzheimers Dement 2014; 10(3): 372-80.
[http://dx.doi.org/10.1016/j.jalz.2013.11.003] [PMID: 24589433]

[9]   Alzheimer's A. 2015 Alzheimer's disease facts and figures. Alzheimers Dement 2015; 11(3): 332-84.
[http://dx.doi.org/10.1016/j.jalz.2015.02.003] [PMID: 25984581]

[10]   Hardy J, Selkoe DJ. The amyloid hypothesis of Alzheimer's disease: progress and problems on the road to therapeutics. Science 2002; 297(5580): 353-6.
[http://dx.doi.org/10.1126/science.1072994] [PMID: 12130773]

[11]   Armstrong RA. A critical analysis of the 'amyloid cascade hypothesis'. Folia Neuropathol 2014; 52(3): 211-25.
[http://dx.doi.org/10.5114/fn.2014.45562] [PMID: 25310732]

[12]   Bishop NA, Lu T, Yankner BA. Neural mechanisms of ageing and cognitive decline. Nature 2010;

464(7288): 529-35.
[http://dx.doi.org/10.1038/nature08983] [PMID: 20336135]

[13]　Hardy J, Selkoe DJ. The amyloid hypothesis of Alzheimer's disease: progress and problems on the road to therapeutics. Science 2002; 297(5580): 353-6.
[http://dx.doi.org/10.1126/science.1072994] [PMID: 12130773]

[14]　Higuchi M, Iwata N, Saido TC. Understanding molecular mechanisms of proteolysis in Alzheimer's disease: progress toward therapeutic interventions. Biochim Biophys Acta 2005; 1751(1): 60-7.
[http://dx.doi.org/10.1016/j.bbapap.2005.02.013] [PMID: 16054018]

[15]　Deane RJ. Is RAGE still a therapeutic target for Alzheimer's disease? Future Med Chem 2012; 4(7): 915-25.
[http://dx.doi.org/10.4155/fmc.12.51] [PMID: 22571615]

[16]　Baranello RJ, Bharani KL, Padmaraju V, *et al.* Amyloid-beta protein clearance and degradation (ABCD) pathways and their role in Alzheimer's disease. Curr Alzheimer Res 2015; 12(1): 32-46.
[http://dx.doi.org/10.2174/1567205012666141218140953] [PMID: 25523424]

[17]　Nalivaeva NN, Fisk LR, Belyaev ND, Turner AJ. Amyloid-degrading enzymes as therapeutic targets in Alzheimer's disease. Curr Alzheimer Res 2008; 5(2): 212-24.
[http://dx.doi.org/10.2174/156720508783954785] [PMID: 18393806]

[18]　Higuchi M, Iwata N, Saido TC. Understanding molecular mechanisms of proteolysis in Alzheimer's disease: progress toward therapeutic interventions. Biochim Biophys Acta 2005; 1751(1): 60-7.
[http://dx.doi.org/10.1016/j.bbapap.2005.02.013] [PMID: 16054018]

[19]　Deane RJ. Is RAGE still a therapeutic target for Alzheimer's disease? Future Med Chem 2012; 4(7): 915-25.
[http://dx.doi.org/10.4155/fmc.12.51] [PMID: 22571615]

[20]　Baranello RJ, Bharani KL, Padmaraju V, *et al.* Amyloid-beta protein clearance and degradation (ABCD) pathways and their role in Alzheimer's disease. Curr Alzheimer Res 2015; 12(1): 32-46.
[http://dx.doi.org/10.2174/1567205012666141218140953] [PMID: 25523424]

[21]　Güell-Bosch J, Montoliu-Gaya L, Esquerda-Canals G, Villegas S. Aβ immunotherapy for Alzheimer's disease: where are we? Neurodegener Dis Manag 2016; 6(3): 179-81.
[http://dx.doi.org/10.2217/nmt-2016-0006] [PMID: 27230296]

[22]　Bates KA, Verdile G, Li QX, *et al.* Clearance mechanisms of Alzheimer's amyloid-beta peptide: implications for therapeutic design and diagnostic tests. Mol Psychiatry 2009; 14(5): 469-86.
[http://dx.doi.org/10.1038/mp.2008.96] [PMID: 18794889]

[23]　Ferreira ST, Clarke JR, Bomfim TR, De Felice FG. Inflammation, defective insulin signaling, and neuronal dysfunction in Alzheimer's disease. Alzheimers Dement 2014; 10(1) (Suppl.): S76-83.
[http://dx.doi.org/10.1016/j.jalz.2013.12.010] [PMID: 24529528]

[24]　Zhang S, Zhang L, Sun A, Jiang H, Qian J, Ge J. Efficacy of statin therapy in chronic systolic cardiac insufficiency: a meta-analysis. Eur J Intern Med 2011; 22(5): 478-84.
[http://dx.doi.org/10.1016/j.ejim.2011.06.003] [PMID: 21925056]

[25]　Golde TE. Overcoming translational barriers impeding development of Alzheimer's disease modifying therapies. J Neurochem 2016; 139 (Suppl. 2): 224-36.
[http://dx.doi.org/10.1111/jnc.13583] [PMID: 27145445]

[26]　Panza F, Frisardi V, Solfrizzi V, *et al.* Immunotherapy for Alzheimer's disease: from anti-β-amyloid to tau-based immunization strategies. Immunotherapy 2012; 4(2): 213-38.
[http://dx.doi.org/10.2217/imt.11.170] [PMID: 22339463]

[27]　Li Y, Liu Y, Wang Z, Jiang Y. Clinical trials of amyloid-based immunotherapy for Alzheimer's disease: end of beginning or beginning of end? Expert Opin Biol Ther 2013; 13(11): 1515-22.
[http://dx.doi.org/10.1517/14712598.2013.838555] [PMID: 24053611]

[28]   Le Couteur DG, Hunter S, Brayne C. Solanezumab and the amyloid hypothesis for Alzheimer's disease. BMJ 2016; 355: i6771.
[http://dx.doi.org/10.1136/bmj.i6771] [PMID: 28034844]

[29]   Wiessner C, Wiederhold KH, Tissot AC, *et al*. The second-generation active Aβ immunotherapy CAD106 reduces amyloid accumulation in APP transgenic mice while minimizing potential side effects. J Neurosci 2011; 31(25): 9323-31.
[http://dx.doi.org/10.1523/JNEUROSCI.0293-11.2011] [PMID: 21697382]

[30]   Ryan JM, Grundman M. Anti-amyloid-beta immunotherapy in Alzheimer's disease: ACC-001 clinical trials are ongoing. J Alzheimers Dis 2009; 17(2): 243.
[http://dx.doi.org/10.3233/JAD-2009-1118] [PMID: 19502708]

[31]   Tayeb HO, Murray ED, Price BH, Tarazi FI. Bapineuzumab and solanezumab for Alzheimer's disease: is the 'amyloid cascade hypothesis' still alive? Expert Opin Biol Ther 2013; 13(7): 1075-84.
[http://dx.doi.org/10.1517/14712598.2013.789856] [PMID: 23574434]

[32]   Sevigny J, Chiao P, Bussière T, *et al*. The antibody aducanumab reduces Aβ plaques in Alzheimer's disease. Nature 2016; 537(7618): 50-6.
[http://dx.doi.org/10.1038/nature19323] [PMID: 27582220]

[33]   Panza F, Seripa D, Solfrizzi V, *et al*. Emerging drugs to reduce abnormal β-amyloid protein in Alzheimer's disease patients. Expert Opin Emerg Drugs 2016; 21(4): 377-91. [Review].
[http://dx.doi.org/10.1080/14728214.2016.1241232] [PMID: 27678025]

[34]   De Strooper B. Lessons from a failed γ-secretase Alzheimer trial. Cell 2014; 159(4): 721-6.
[http://dx.doi.org/10.1016/j.cell.2014.10.016] [PMID: 25417150]

[35]   Matthew E Kennedy. The BACE1 inhibitor verubecestat (MK-8931) reduces CNS b-amyloid in animal models and in Alzheimer's disease patients. Sci Transl Med 2016; 8(363): 363ra150.

[36]   Braak H, Braak E. 1996; Evolution of the neuropathology of Alzheimer's disease. Acta Neurol Scand 1996; 165(Suppl): 3-12.
[http://dx.doi.org/10.1111/j.1600-0404.1996.tb05866.x]

[37]   Nelson PT, Alafuzoff I, Bigio EH, *et al*. Correlation of Alzheimer disease neuropathologic changes with cognitive status: a review of the literature. J Neuropathol Exp Neurol 2012; 71(5): 362-81.
[http://dx.doi.org/10.1097/NEN.0b013e31825018f7] [PMID: 22487856]

[38]   Braak E, Griffing K, Arai K, Bohl J, Bratzke H, Braak H. Neuropathology of Alzheimer's disease: what is new since A. Alzheimer? Eur Arch Psychiatry Clin Neurosci 1999; 249 (Suppl. 3): 14-22.
[http://dx.doi.org/10.1007/PL00014168] [PMID: 10654095]

[39]   Morris M, Maeda S, Vossel K, Mucke L. The many faces of tau. Neuron 2011; 70(3): 410-26.
[http://dx.doi.org/10.1016/j.neuron.2011.04.009] [PMID: 21555069]

[40]   Underwood E. NEUROSCIENCE. Alzheimer's amyloid theory gets modest boost. Science 2015; 349(6247): 464.
[http://dx.doi.org/10.1126/science.349.6247.464] [PMID: 26228122]

[41]   Johnell K, Fastbom J. Concurrent use of anticholinergic drugs and cholinesterase inhibitors: register-based study of over 700,000 elderly patients. Drugs Aging 2008; 25(10): 871-7.
[http://dx.doi.org/10.2165/00002512-200825100-00006] [PMID: 18808211]

[42]   Stuck AE, Siu AL, Wieland GD, Adams J, Rubenstein LZ. Comprehensive geriatric assessment: a meta-analysis of controlled trials. Lancet 1993; 342(8878): 1032-6.
[http://dx.doi.org/10.1016/0140-6736(93)92884-V] [PMID: 8105269]

[43]   Haas M, Mantua V, Haberkamp M, *et al*. The European Medicines Agency's strategies to meet the challenges of Alzheimer disease. Nat Rev Drug Discov 2015; 14(4): 221-2.
[http://dx.doi.org/10.1038/nrd4585] [PMID: 25829266]

[44]   Winblad B, Amouyel P, Andrieu S, *et al*. Defeating Alzheimer's disease and other dementias: a

priority for European science and society. Lancet Neurol 2016; 15(5): 455-532.
[http://dx.doi.org/10.1016/S1474-4422(16)00062-4] [PMID: 26987701]

[45]   Canter RG, Penney J, Tsai LH. The road to restoring neural circuits for the treatment of Alzheimer's disease. Nature 2016; 539(7628): 187-96.
[http://dx.doi.org/10.1038/nature20412] [PMID: 27830780]

CHAPTER 2

Brain Connectivity in Alzheimer's Disease: From the Disconnection Syndrome to the Search for New Biomarkers

Alberto Marcos Dolado[*], David López Sanz, María Eugenia López García, Miguel Yus Fuertes, Laura Marcos Arribas, Cristina López Mico and **Fernando Maestú Unturbe**

Neurology Department, Hospital Clinico San Carlos, Madrid, Spain

Abstract: In recent years, the research of Alzheimer's disease (AD) has shifted from the classic paradigm of grey matter disorders as the central and most relevant events of the pathophysiology, to a broader perspective that takes into account the role of white matter and brain connectivity. In the pre-AD stage, the mild cognitive impairment, we can find with Magnetoencephalography a pattern of desynchronization among some regions related with brain disconnection and hyper synchronization probably as a compensatory mechanism. In addition, the study of brain white matter tracts by diffusion tensor imaging by MRI provides sufficient discriminative capacity to allow its use in the prognosis of the evolution of subjects within early stages of the disease. Along these lines, we expect to show the alterations of white matter tracts in early phases of the disease, and the possibility of using them as a predictor of the development of AD. The study of connectivity alterations not only allows us to know the physio pathogenic basis of the disease but also to increase targets in the search for earlier markers of this neurodegenerative disorder.

Keywords: Alzheimer's Disease, Mild Cognitive Impairment, Preclinical Stages, Fractional Anisotropy, Mean Diffusivity, Diffusion Tensor Imaging, Brain connectivity, Early biomarker.

INTRODUCTION

Dementia is one of the most devastating diseases in developed countries. Alzheimer's Disease (AD) is the most frequent cause of dementia in our environment. Its incidence and prevalence grow exponentially with age, implying a significant public health problem. By the beginning of this century, 4.6 million new AD cases were diagnosed every year all over the world [1]. The increase

[*] **Corresponding author Alberto Marcos Dolado:** Department of Neurology, Hospital Clinico San Carlos, C/ Martin Lagos s/n, 28040, Madrid, Spain; Tel: +34630954013; E-mail: amarcosdolado@gmail.com

Blas Gil-Extremera (Ed.)

in life expectancy comes at a cost, as AD rates are expected to dramatically grow in the following years. Around 2025, almost every state in the US is prone to experience a double to triple-digit percentage increase in AD prevalence [2]. Given the economic and social cost of AD in the near future, its early diagnosis and treatment represent a major challenge for modern science.

This progressive neurodegenerative disorder is of unknown aetiology, but abnormal deposits and protein malfunctions have been implicated. Classically, neuronal loss, formation of extracellular beta-amyloid plaques and intracyto-plasmic neurofibrillary tangles of hyper phosphorylated tau protein [3, 4] have been the main hallmarks. These pathological accumulations occur in different locations of the cerebral cortex, being more frequent in the entorhinal cortex and in the hippocampus. These alterations observed in pathological samples or through neuroimaging are one of its main diagnostic criteria. However, outside research environments, the diagnosis is usually based on the patient's clinical profile, which is varied and responds to a deterioration of cognitive functions. The most common intellective alteration is usually memory impairment, especially episodic and, later on, semantic and procedural. Executive or visuospatial decline may also occur, together with any other psychiatric symptoms, either from early stages but especially during the progression of the disease [3]. Although until recently, patients were diagnosed when dementia was beginning, in the last decades, the use of biomarkers has diverted the diagnostic approach to phases prior to the development of functional limitations. Clinical concepts, such as Mild Cognitive Impairment (MCI) due to AD, Subjective Cognitive Decline (SCD) or even presymptomatic stages, have been introduced, which have triggered the need to find new biomarkers, along with neuroimaging studies and neuropsychological tests [4, 5].

IMAGE BASED DIAGNOSIS

Neuroimaging findings may be useful to rule out other pathologies or to support the diagnosis, but the majority of lesions observed are non-specific to AD and may be found in other dementias or in the aging brain. Macroscopically, in AD there is marked atrophy of the hippocampi, the parahippocampal convolutions and temporal, parietal and frontal lobes. Structural neuroimaging has shown an ability to identify those MCI that progress to AD with a sensitivity of 73% and a specificity of 81% but only using volumetric techniques, which are not readily available and require extended study times [6]. The two most validated techniques that are currently available for the specific diagnosis of AD are the Amyloid-Positron Emission Tomography (PET) and the 2-deoxy-2-[fluorine-18]fluro-D-glucose integrated with computed tomography (FDG-PET). The PiB-PET allows measuring the volume of lesions by detecting the density of amyloid plaques, helping not only diagnosis and prognosis but also the development of drugs that interact with amyloid deposits. An important inconvenience is that it is rarely available in most clinics, it depends on an experienced examiner and has a very high cost. FDG-PET shows areas of hypometabolism in the hippocampus, precuneus and lateral parietal and posterior temporal cortex regions. The discriminatory capacity of FDG-PET to differentiate AD from other forms of dementia in autopsy confirmed studies was close to 90% in sensitivity and 80% in specificity [6]. But it is also unavailable in many settings outside research studies and offers no information in the very early stages.

OTHER BIOMARKERS

Cerebrospinal fluid amyloid beta ($A\beta42$) levels predicted conversion from MCI to AD with 60–80% sensitivity and 65–100% specificity, and total-tau (t-tau) levels 83–86% sensitivity and 56–90% specificity. Nevertheless, there are significant differences among studies with considerable inter-site assay variability. Additionally, it is an invasive and non-risk-free technique that requires centralized laboratories that are not available in many cities. Furthermore, the presence of one or two alleles of the apolipoprotein E (ApoE) 4 genotype appears to increase the risk of developing AD in non-demented patients and MCI patients, being appropriate in presymptomatic research studies and in clinical trials but not in routine practice.

Finally, due to its accessibility and low cost, the most extended diagnostic markers in the specialized examination are the neuropsychological tests. Cognitive exploration is quite useful to evaluate patients with SCD or MCI, whose diagnosis corresponds to transitional states between normal cognition and dementia with daily living activities not affected. Neuropsychology has proofed discriminative capacity to determine the risk of progression from MCI to AD, although its validity to differentiate between normal aging and other psycho-affective processes is not determined [7].

But much of the limitations we currently have to detect AD in the predementia phase are probably due to the antiquated nosological concept of the entity. Traditionally, brain processes and cognitive abilities have been associated to specific brain regions. This conception of brain functioning, the so-called *localizationism*, is mainly supported by the study of the consequences on specific cognitive functions produced by focal brain abnormalities. However, the unprecedented development of brain imaging techniques is allowing a better understanding of brain functioning, being now considered as a complex network in which different brain regions are involved in cognition. Thus, in recent years, the research of AD has shifted from the classic paradigm of grey matter disorders to a broader perspective that takes into account the role of white matter and brain connectivity. These advances have fostered the idea that successful brain processing comes from distributed and synchronized activity in multiple brain areas, a concept known as *functional connectivity* (FC). Besides, this measure may be used with the data obtained from different imaging techniques, such as electroencephalography (EEG), magnetoencephalography (MEG), functional magnetic resonance imaging (fMRI) or PET, making it an utterly useful and flexible tool. In fact, both the International Working Group and the American Alzheimer's Association have recently highlighted the promising perspective of FC as an early biomarker of AD, even at its preclinical stages [8].

ALZHEIMER'S DISEASE AS A DISCONNECTION SYNDROME

The disruption of the communication between different brain regions has been a common finding in AD. One of the networks that has been most described as altered is the Resting State Network (RSN), a set of interacting brain regions known to have a highly correlated activity with others and that are activated "by default" when a person is not focused on the outside world, but when he thinks of himself, remembering the past or imagining the future [9]. The RSN involves important roles in episodic memory [10] executive control and monitoring [11], that are even detectable during some sleep stages [12]. In AD changes have been described in the normal FC brain pattern during resting state [13, 14] and also while executing a cognitive task [15]. In fact, AD pathology impairs neuronal synapses through different mechanisms, thus limiting the normal brain temporal coordination. Consequently, AD has been conceptualized as a *disconnection syndrome* [16]. Several neuroimaging studies have revealed a decrease in FC in AD compared to healthy controls. The functional coupling between bilateral hippocampi and several brain regions involving frontal, parietal, temporal and occipital lobes is diminished in AD patients [13, 14]. One of the topics capturing more attention nowadays in AD is how its pathology affects the different RSNs. These groups of inter-connected brain areas tend to be stable across healthy individuals, thus allowing their identification as a result of their specific spatio-temporal patterns [17].

One of the RSNs that is currently gaining more attention for its prominent role in the AD continuum is the Default Mode Network (DMN), which comprises medial prefrontal cortices, bilateral inferior parietal lobules, medial temporal structures, such as the hippocampus, and particularly the precuneus/posterior cingulate cortex (PCC). This latter region is a crucial structure within this network and is commonly considered as a hub for DMN connectivity analysis. DMN areas are known to be highly connected in wakeful resting state, while dampening their coupling whenever the subject engages in a cognitive task [18]. It has been revealed that the DMN connectivity is consistently disrupted in AD patients. A number of studies have addressed DMN synchronization by placing a *seed* in the PCC (*i.e.* measuring the connectivity of this region with other brain areas) finding a decreased connectivity in frontal, parietal and also PCC regions in AD patients [19]. Combining functional MRI, FC and structural connectivity (SC) measured by Tensor Diffusion Imaging (DTI), Soldner and colleagues [20] reported significant damage in early AD stages in a critical pathway for DMN communication that connects PCC and hippocampus through parahippocampal gyrus. Additionally, the spatial pattern of β-amyloid accumulation in AD has been closely linked to key regions of the DMN, such as precuneus or PCC [21]. Furthermore, β-amyloid accumulation in AD related areas predicts a greater disconnection over posterior DMN areas such as the inferior parietal lobe [22]. Those findings altogether highlight the relevance of the application of FC in specific brain networks, such as the DMN, during the course of AD.

Besides seed-based analysis, one of the most common means to study FC is Independent Component Analysis (ICA). This algorithm seeks to identify the underlying statistically independent components of the brain activation. As a result, brain networks can be identified and segregated from each other in a data-driven manner. It is not an uncommon way of identifying fractioned versions of traditional RSNs into their spatial subcomponents by using ICA analysis. For instance, the DMN is usually split into anterior (aDMN) and posterior (pDMN) subcomponents, or even into more subdivisions [23]. Thanks to this method, recent studies have found that different subcomponents of the DMN are affected differently along the AD continuum. In his study, Damoiseaux [24] reported a progressive synchronization decrease in the anterior as well as the posterior components of the DMN in healthy elders. Studies have shown that FC decreases in pDMN were larger in patients with AD compared to healthy elders, while the aDMN exhibited hyper synchronization in the patient group. This was interpreted as a prolonged inefficiency in the brain of those individuals affected by AD pathology [25]. Interestingly, recent studies suggest that the trajectory of FC disruption in AD might not be linear, and the direction of the alterations observed in different stages of the disease could change, providing a means of disease severity. According to these studies, synchronization in aDMN is increased in the early stages of the disease while the pDMN component seems to be reduced. However, in later stages, once AD becomes more severe, connectivity in all subsystems is progressively dampened, reducing their synchronization compared to healthy controls. Increases in FC in AD patients described in the literature have been commonly interpreted as a compensatory mechanism [21]. According to this compensatory hypothesis, those brain networks affected by AD pathology would increase their level of activation or synchronicity beyond normal levels in an effort to successfully overcome the demands of a certain task or situation.

However, a recent work points out that this hyper-excitability, on the contrary, may represent a pathological feature of the disease, reflecting inefficient or noisy information processing by the brain [26]. Furthermore, it has been proposed that this processing burden could be propagated through downstream highly connected nodes along brain networks, thus spreading the disease and provoking a cascading network failure in AD patients. In the same vein, the nodal stress hypothesis predicts that an increase in metabolic demands in key hubs for information flow would, in turn, increase nodal vulnerability, worsening the atrophy level of those regions [27].

THE APPROACH IN THE EARLY STAGES OF THE DISEASE

It is noteworthy that prodromal stages of AD may start up to 10 or even 15 years before clinical diagnosis [28]. As a consequence, many studies are focusing on identifying brain signatures of AD pathology before clinical symptoms become evident. MCI represents an at-risk state for developing dementia, in which patients suffer a mild decline in one or more cognitive domains. The annual conversion rate from MCI to AD has been estimated around 8% to 15% [29]. Curiously, several studies have already demonstrated that MCI patients already exhibit FC alterations, sharing some similarities with those observed in AD. In a recent study reconstructing source space FC with MEG, the MCI group showed reduced mean synchronization in pDMN regions in the alpha frequency band [30] as previously described in both FC and SC findings [31]. Furthermore, when comparing whole brain connectivity to healthy control elders, synchronization in the MCI group was significantly reduced over a widespread posterior network comprising occipital, parietal, as well as medial and lateral temporal structures, such as hippocampus, a critical region closely linked to the initial stages of the disease. In contrast, synchronization over frontal regions, including the anterior cingulate cortex and medial frontal gyrus, was increased in MCI with respect to healthy elders. This dual pattern of anterior hyper synchronization and posterior desynchronization in resting state is consistent with the findings obtained in AD patients and has been replicated in different MCI samples. Along the same line, Canuet [32] described in a MCI sample a decrement in connectivity mainly over posterior and temporal areas and an increment in anterior areas, which were related to the concentration of CSF biomarkers (phospho-tau and amyloid). Additionally, these connectivity alterations have been explored by network measures derived from the Minimum Spanning Tree (MST) revealing that MCI brain functioning seems to be more inefficient than those of the healthy elders [33]. Several resting state studies exploring the progression from MCI to AD have reported differences in synchronization between those MCIs that remain stable (sMCI) and those that finally progress to dementia (pMCI). Although some resting state studies have failed to find functional connectivity differences between MCI and healthy controls [34, 35], most have shown an increase in low-frequency activity, which has been usually accompanied by a decrease in synchronization. For example, in MCI subjects, Moretti [36] reported an intra-hemispheric fronto-parietal decline coherence with a temporal inter-hemispheric increase when compared to elderly controls, and Gómez [37] found a decrease in beta band synchronization. From our group, López [38], in two years' follow-up study, found that pMCI exhibited hyper synchronization between anterior cingulate and posterior brain structures compared to sMCI. Comparing 30 sMCI and 19 pMCI subjects and correlating with neuropsychological scores and entorhinal, parahippocampal, and hippocampal volumes, pMCI patients obtained lower scores in episodic and semantic memory and executive functioning. The pMCI patients group exhibited a higher synchronization than sMCI subjects in the alpha band between the right anterior cingulate and temporo-occipital regions. This hyper synchronization was inversely correlated with cognitive performance and both hippocampal volumes being predictive of conversion from MCI to AD. The combined power predicting progression to AD of both neuropsychological and neurophysiological data achieves an accuracy of 89.8% (95% CI:77.8–96.6%, 89.5% sensitivity, 90.0% specificity, 85.0% positive predictive value, 93.1% negative predictive value), greater than if these two variables were considered separately. Interestingly, there were no differences in hippocampal volume between groups, indicating that this biomarker, one of the most commonly used, would not have offered discriminative value of the evolution in this cohort.

But we can approach the study of the FC beyond the domain of brain resting. If we estimate connectivity parameters during the performance of specific tasks we will find significant differences in the function of brain state. Short term memory activities increased interhemispheric synchronization in most frequency bands and higher connectivity between temporo-frontal regions in pMCIs when compared to healthy people [39, 40]. Mental calculation abilities are commonly impaired early in the course of AD. Its deterioration correlates with glucose hypometabolism in the left inferior parietal lobule, left inferior temporal gyrus and prefrontal regions. Although simple calculation is preserved in MCI, early problems appear when inhibition processes are required [41].

In this area, our group studied a combination between resting state and a cognitive state with no external stimuli, a condition named "Internally Directed Cognitive State" in 34 healthy elders and 55 MCI patients [42]. Compared to the control group, MCI patients presented higher connectivity values, together with a lower cognitive performance, in most bands with a lack of synchronization in the alpha band, which may denote an inhibitory deficit. The increased connectivity between the left and right anterior regions highlights the necessity of the interaction between both hemispheres for the performance of mental calculation. Furthermore, the increase in functional connectivity seems to be a compensatory mechanism prior to definitive claudication and loss of brain efficiency [43]. The anterior regions of the DMN were found to be more desynchronized in the control group, indicating that MCIs were not able to sufficiently deactivate this network to perform the task. We also have enough data to believe that this profile of hyper synchronization in the MCI may be related to the pathological process of AD. Correlations have been described between hyperactivity, neuronal hyper excitability and the release of beta amyloid protein into interstitial fluid, with greater excitability leading to greater neuronal synchronization [44 - 46].

Although the nosological concept of MCI still raises some controversy, the current classification of its subtypes according to the affected domains has great utility in the evolutionary prognosis [47, 48]. In a recent study [49] with 105 subjects (36 healthy controls, 33 amnestic single domain MCIs, a-sd-MCI, and 36 amnestic multidomain MCIs, a-md-MCI) we found, in the a-md-MCI group, a significant power increase within delta and theta ranges and reduced relative power within alpha and beta ranges, showing this subtype not only a slowing of the spectrum but also ~~with~~ a poorer cognitive status, close to that observed in AD. In the same way Fernandez [50] demonstrated that an increase in delta activity in posterior regions such as the right posterior parietal cortex and the precuneus indexed the transition from MCI to mild and from mild to more severe dementia with a 3.5-fold increase in conversion risk. A-md-MCI patients combined with exaggerated delta and theta activity seem to adequately represent prodromal AD. We also recently found [51] that the combination of structural measures (left hippocampal volume), MEG measurements (occipital cortex theta power), and neuropsychological scores predicted conversion of 33 MCI patients to AD with 100% sensitivity and 94.7% specificity.

If we look at even earlier phases in the spectrum of AD, the SCD represents an asymptomatic group of elders presenting a subjective feeling of cognitive worsening but with normal range in standard neuropsychological assessment and daily living performance [52]. A growing number of studies highlight increased conversion rates to AD in this population, compared to control elders [53]. Moreover, characteristic AD features have also been observed in their brain activity [54] and CSF [55]. Furthermore, there are studies reporting a similar FC pattern of alterations that found in MCI [30], with an anterior increase and a posterior decrease in FC, affecting DMN regions among others (Fig. **1**). Interestingly, it was also shown that this population exhibited similar alterations to those of MCI patients in their spectral properties [54] and their network topology [56]. However, this entity has been scarcely studied, and further clinical, pathological and resting state functional connectivity investigations may provide relevant information in order to better understand whether it should be included as a preclinical stage of the AD continuum.

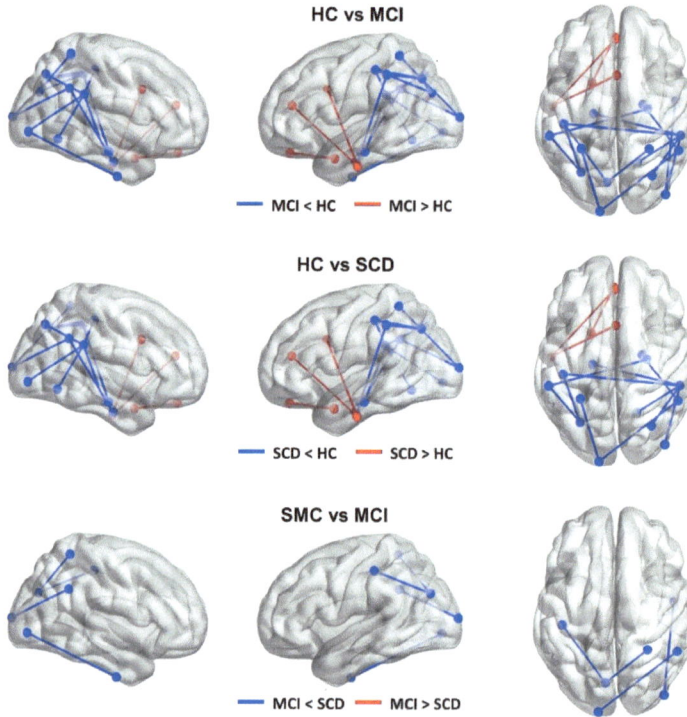

Fig. (1). The figure shows differences in Functional Connectivity (FC) between groups. Blue lines indicate desynchronization in the group in the more advanced stage of the disease. On the contrary, red lines indicate an increase in FC in this group. HC= Healthy controls; MCI= Mild Cognitive Impairment; SCD=Subjective Cognitive Decline.

Another great current tool for measuring brain connectivity is the Diffusion Tensor Imaging (DTI) technique. MRI plus DTI offers a non-invasive means with adequate capacity for spatial discrimination to examine the distribution of the white matter tracts and their anatomical integrity. DTI characterizes the three-dimensional diffusion of water in its spatial location within the white matter tracts using mainly two parameters: Mean Diffusivity (MD), which describes the rotationally invariant magnitude of water diffusion, and Fractional Anisotropy (FA), a measure indicating its overall directionality. Some authors [57, 58] have found connectivity variations between MCI, AD and controls, while others have not corroborated it [59], or found methodological problems [60].

Considering the contradictory results, we included 217 subjects, ranging from age 65 to 80, and at different clinical stages (70 controls, 126 MCI and 21 AD). After they underwent neuropsychological testing and a DTI scan, MD and FA of several tracts was estimated in order to discriminate multiple brain networks as prognostic markers of progression from the early to the dementia stage of AD [61]. Neuropsychological testing was repeated every 6 months in both patients and controls. MR images were acquired using a 1.5 Tesla scanner (General Electric Medical Systems, Waukesha, WI) with HDxt release 16.0 and an eight-channel, high-resolution head coil. In addition to whole head 3D fast spoiled gradient-echo T1-weighted 1 mm^3 isotropic sequence, 3D CUBE FLAIR T2-weighted 1.6 mm thickness sequence and 2D gradient-echo T2 sequences, DTI images were also obtained. After registration to standard space MNI1552 (Fig. **2**), FA and MD maps were generated. We can see in Table **1**, the initial values of FA and MD in the different areas in the whole group. In 40 months of median follow-up, 80 MCI patients remained stable, while 46 developed AD criteria, with a conversion rate of 36,5%. In the sensitivity and specificity study, the alteration shown in some tracts, such as the left uncinate fasciculus, the right cingulum and the left parahippocampal white matter, are able to predict the progression from MCI to AD and, therefore, they are liable to be used as early diagnostic tools. We show in Table **2**, the cut-off points chosen for maximum sensitivities and specificities for those tracts whose Area Under the Curve (AUC) was estimated to be relevant (AUC> 0.55, p <0.05). As can be seen, the mean value of FA in the different tracts is higher in non-converters than in the converters group. A logistic regression study was conducted in order to select the variables that present the greatest predictive capacity for progression from MCI to AD. No MD or neuropsychological value reached significance. The resulting variables are shown in Table **3**. A direct relationship between the increase in FA in the left uncinated fascicle and the dementia risk is observed. Conversely, in the right cingulum and left parahippocampal white matter, as the FA decreases, the probability of conversion increases. Various explanations might apply, but we postulate that both the right cingulum and the left parahippocampal white matter may play a compensatory role in the evolution to dementia, trying to account for the loss of connectivity in other areas, increasing their functionality until later stages of the disease, in which successive aggressions would cause their claudication.

Table 1. Fractional Anisotrophy and Mean Diffusivity of selected areas.

Imaging areas	AUC	CI (95%)	p
Callosum FA	0,634	0,536-0,732	0,015
R cingulum FA	0,666	0,574-0,759	0,003
L cingulum FA	0,692	0,602-0,782	0,001
R uncinate FA	0,616	0,521-0,712	0,036
L uncinate FA	0,559	0,457-0,661	0,288
R hippocampal FA	0,694	0,602-0,787	0,000

(Table 1) cont.....

Imaging areas	AUC	CI (95%)	p
L hippocampal FA	0,681	0,585-0,777	0,001
Callosum MD	0,550	0,447-0,653	0,370
R cingulum MD	0,579	0,478-0,681	0,150
L cingulum MD	0,560	0,456-0,664	0,275
R uncinate MD	0,537	0,438-0,636	0,501
L uncinate MD	0,543	0,441-0,645	0,437
R hippocampal MD	0,588	0,490-0,685	0,112
L hippocampal MD	0,621	0,531-0,711	0,028

FA: Fractional anisotrophy; MD: Mean diffusivity; AUC: Area under the curve; CI: Confidence interval; R: Right; L: Left.

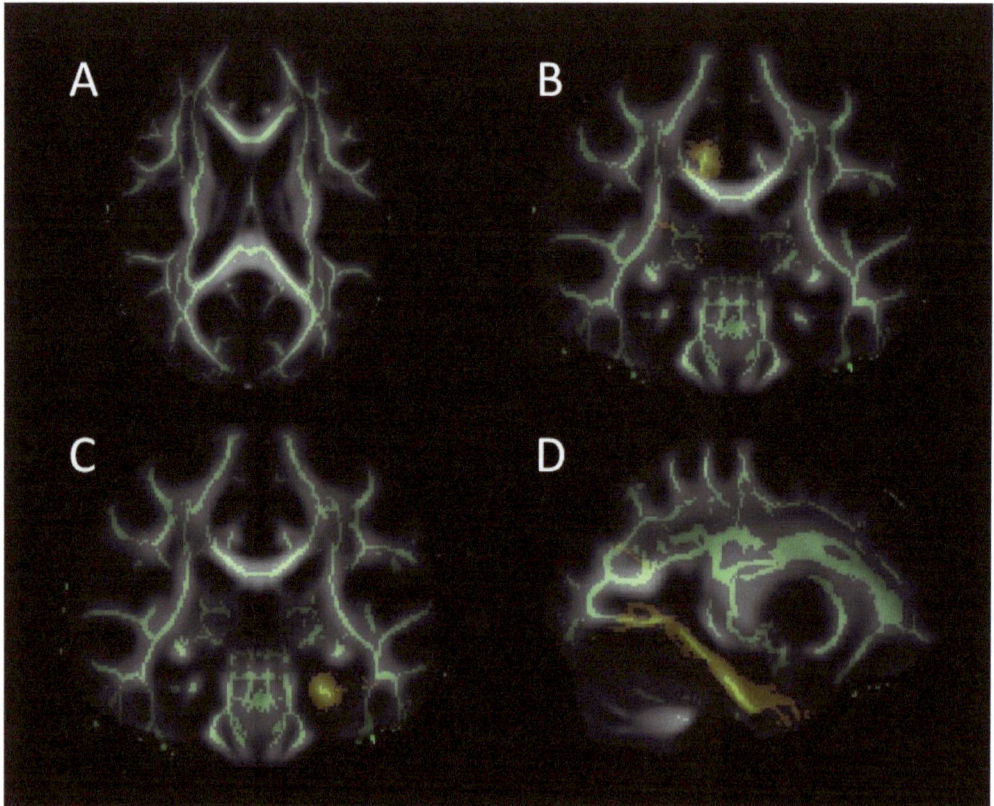

Fig. (2). FMRIB58 image (resulting from the fractional anisotropy map average of 58 healthy subjects after registration to standard space MNI1552) with overlap (in green) from the projection to an average skeletal representation representing the spatial centers of all the tracts common to group (A). Mask overlap (yellow) corresponding to areas of the white matter tractographic atlas JHU corresponding to the right cingulum (B), and left hippocampus (C, D), probabilistically identified after probabilistic tractography and used for the extraction of regional data of the value of FA of each subject.

Table 2. Cut points with greater sensitivity and specificity and means for the FA and MD measurements with AUC> 0.55.

Tracts	Cut point	Sensibility	1-Specificity	Converters mean	Non converters mean
Callosum FA	0,55431	0,714	0,477	0,54282	0,55345
R cingulum FA	0,47911	0,743	0,445	0,46740	0,48762
L cingulum FA	0,48277	0,800	0,438	0,47066	0,48971
R uncinate FA	0,41821	0,686	0,453	0,41305	0,43238
L uncinate FA	0,55149	0,600	0,438	0,42169	0,42903
R hippocampus FA	0,48372	0,800	0,461	0,46573	0,48789
L hippocampus FA	0,4474	0,743	0,438	0,43296	0,45890
L hippocampus MD	0,00082	0,743	0,602	0,04996	0,08942

FA: Fractional anisotrophy; MD: Mean diffusivity; AUC: Area under the curve; CI: Confidence interval; R: Right; L: Left.

Table 3. Significant tracts values after logistic regression.

Tracts	Value	SD	p
R cingulum FA	-21,834	9,922	0,028
L uncinate FA	19,787	6,746	0,003
L hippocampus FA	-20,073	8,020	0,012

FA: Fractional anisotrophy; MD: Mean diffusivity; SD: Standart deviation; R: Right; L: Left.

FROM THE REVISED NOSOLOGICAL CONCEPT TO THE SEARCH OF NEW BIOMARKERS

In summary, AD has been classically defined as a grey matter disease. Nevertheless, amyloid deposits and neuronal destruction are not able to fully explain the whole pathophysiology of AD. It is for this reason, together with the aforementioned evidence, that the disconnection hypothesis has been postulated, also giving importance to the involvement of the white matter tracts that join the different neuronal nuclei. The study of connectivity alterations not only allows to characterize the physiopathogenic basis of the disease but also to increase targets in the search for early markers of the disease. In the prodromal-AD stage, namely MCI, a dual pattern coexists: on one hand, the desynchronization, related with brain disconnection, and on the other hand, the hyper synchronization, that may be interpreted as a compensatory mechanism or as an aberrant functioning. On the whole, these synchronization/desynchronization profiles measured by MEG spectral mapping seem to be a serious candidate as a marker of dysfunctional synaptic transmission in the disease, and in some cases superior to conventional structural imaging as a predictor of progression to dementia. In addition, the study of brain white matter tracts by DTI provides sufficient discriminative capacity to allow its use in the prognosis of the evolution of subjects with early stages of AD in the specialized clinical setting.

We sought to convey that the alterations of white matter tracts that occur early in the most devastating neurodegenerative disease of our time and the possibility of using these changes as a predictor of the evolution allow us to early detect AD and also alter the nosological concept of the entity.

CONCLUSIONS

1.- Although AD has been classically defined as a grey matter disease, large evidence indicates an important pathogenic role of the disconnection of cortical areas caused by white matter lesions.

2.- In the prodromal-AD stages, we found MEG mapping desynchronization related with brain disconnection and hyper synchronization that is interpreted as a compensatory or erroneous mechanism.

3.- These synchronization/desynchronization profiles, measured by MEG mapping, seem to be markers of dysfunctional synaptic transmission in AD and can accurately predict the progression to dementia.

4.- Also, the study of brain white matter tracts by DTI-MRI has sufficient predictive capacity in the prognosis of the evolution to dementia of subjects with early stages of AD.

5.- The study of connectivity not only allows to characterize the pathophysiology of the disease but also the search for early markers.

CONSENT FOR PUBLICATION

Not applicable.

ACKNOWLEDGEMENTS

Project partially funded by the Ministry of Science and Innovation (PSI2009-14415-C03, PSI2012-38375-C03 and PSI2015-68793-C3-R projects).

CONFLICT OF INTEREST

The authors confirm that this chapter contents have no conflict of interest.

REFERENCES

[1]   Ferri CP, Prince M, Brayne C, *et al.* Global prevalence of dementia: a Delphi consensus study. Lancet 2005; 366(9503): 2112-7.
[http://dx.doi.org/10.1016/S0140-6736(05)67889-0] [PMID: 16360788]

[2]   Weuve J, Hebert LE, Scherr PA, Evans DA. Prevalence of Alzheimer disease in US states. Epidemiology 2015; 26(1): e4-6.
[http://dx.doi.org/10.1097/EDE.0000000000000199] [PMID: 25437325]

[3]   Iqbal K, Liu F, Gong CX. Tau and neurodegenerative disease: the story so far. Nat Rev Neurol 2016; 12(1): 15-27.
[http://dx.doi.org/10.1038/nrneurol.2015.225] [PMID: 26635213]

[4]   Reitz C, Mayeux R. Alzheimer disease: epidemiology, diagnostic criteria, risk factors and biomarkers. Biochem Pharmacol 2014; 88(4): 640-51.
[http://dx.doi.org/10.1016/j.bcp.2013.12.024] [PMID: 24398425]

[5]   Fortea J, Vilaplana E, Alcolea D, *et al.* Cerebrospinal fluid β-amyloid and phospho-tau biomarker interactions affecting brain structure in preclinical Alzheimer disease. Ann Neurol 2014; 76(2): 223-30.
[http://dx.doi.org/10.1002/ana.24186] [PMID: 24852682]

[6]   Riverol M, López OL. Biomarkers in Alzheimer's disease. Front Neurol 2011; 2: 46.
[http://dx.doi.org/10.3389/fneur.2011.00046] [PMID: 21808632]

[7]   Marcos A, Gil P, Barabash A, *et al.* Neuropsychological markers of progression from Mild Cognitive Impairment to Alzheimer's disease. Am J Alzheimer dis and other dem 2006; 21(3): 189-96.
[http://dx.doi.org/10.1177/1533317506289348]

[8]   Dubois B, Hampel H, Feldman HH, *et al.* Preclinical Alzheimer's disease: Definition, natural history, and diagnostic criteria. Alzheimers Dement 2016; 12(3): 292-323.
[http://dx.doi.org/10.1016/j.jalz.2016.02.002] [PMID: 27012484]

[9]   Buckner RL, Andrews-Hanna JR, Schacter DL. The brain's default network: anatomy, function, and relevance to disease. Ann N Y Acad Sci 2008; 1124(1): 1-38.
[http://dx.doi.org/10.1196/annals.1440.011] [PMID: 18400922]

[10]   Sami S, Robertson EM, Miall RC. The time course of task-specific memory consolidation effects in resting state networks. J Neurosci 2014; 34(11): 3982-92.
[http://dx.doi.org/10.1523/JNEUROSCI.4341-13.2014] [PMID: 24623776]

[11]   Dong G, Lin X, Potenza MN. Decreased functional connectivity in an executive control network is related to impaired executive function in Internet gaming disorder. Prog Neuropsychopharmacol Biol Psychiatry 2015; 57: 76-85.
[http://dx.doi.org/10.1016/j.pnpbp.2014.10.012] [PMID: 25445475]

[12]   Deco G, Hagmann P, Hudetz AG, Tononi G. Modeling resting-state functional networks when the cortex falls asleep: local and global changes. Cereb Cortex 2014; 24(12): 3180-94.
[http://dx.doi.org/10.1093/cercor/bht176] [PMID: 23845770]

[13]   Allen G, Barnard H, McColl R, *et al.* Reduced hippocampal functional connectivity in Alzheimer disease. Arch Neurol 2007; 64(10): 1482-7.
[http://dx.doi.org/10.1001/archneur.64.10.1482] [PMID: 17923631]

[14]   Wang L, Zang Y, He Y, *et al.* Changes in hippocampal connectivity in the early stages of Alzheimer's disease: evidence from resting state fMRI. Neuroimage 2006; 31(2): 496-504.
[http://dx.doi.org/10.1016/j.neuroimage.2005.12.033] [PMID: 16473024]

[15]   Grady CL, Furey ML, Pietrini P, Horwitz B, Rapoport SI. Altered brain functional connectivity and impaired short-term memory in Alzheimer's disease. Brain 2001; 124(Pt 4): 739-56.
[http://dx.doi.org/10.1093/brain/124.4.739] [PMID: 11287374]

[16]   Bokde ALW, Ewers M, Hampel H. Assessing neuronal networks: understanding Alzheimer's disease. Prog Neurobiol 2009; 89(2): 125-33.
[http://dx.doi.org/10.1016/j.pneurobio.2009.06.004] [PMID: 19560509]

[17]   Damoiseaux JS, Rombouts SARB, Barkhof F, *et al.* Consistent resting-state networks across healthy subjects. Proc Natl Acad Sci USA 2006; 103(37): 13848-53.
[http://dx.doi.org/10.1073/pnas.0601417103] [PMID: 16945915]

[18]   Andrews-Hanna JR, Reidler JS, Huang C, Buckner RL. Evidence for the default network's role in spontaneous cognition. J Neurophysiol 2010; 104(1): 322-35.
[http://dx.doi.org/10.1152/jn.00830.2009] [PMID: 20463201]

[19]   Weiler M, Teixeira CVL, Nogueira MH, *et al.* Differences and the relationship in default mode network intrinsic activity and functional connectivity in mild Alzheimer's disease and amnestic mild cognitive impairment. Brain Connect 2014; 4(8): 567-74.
[http://dx.doi.org/10.1089/brain.2014.0234] [PMID: 25026537]

[20]   Soldner J, Meindl T, Koch W, *et al.* Strukturelle und funktionelle neuronale Konnektivität bei der Alzheimer-Krankheit : Eine kombinierte DTI- und fMRT-Studie. Nervenarzt 2012; 83(7): 878-87.
[http://dx.doi.org/10.1007/s00115-011-3326-3] [PMID: 21713583]

[21]   Mormino EC, Smiljic A, Hayenga AO, *et al.* Relationships between β-amyloid and functional connectivity in different components of the default mode network in aging. Cerebral Cortex (New York, NY : 1991) 2011; 21(10): 2399-407.
[http://dx.doi.org/10.1093/cercor/bhr025]

[22]   Kim HJ, Cha J, Lee JM, *et al.* Distinctive Resting State Network Disruptions Among Alzheimer's Disease, Subcortical Vascular Dementia, and Mixed Dementia Patients. J Alzheimers Dis 2016; 50(3): 709-18.
[http://dx.doi.org/10.3233/JAD-150637] [PMID: 26757039]

[23]   Jones DT, Vemuri P, Murphy MC, *et al.* Non-stationarity in the "resting brain's" modular architecture. PLoS One 2012; 7(6): e39731.
[http://dx.doi.org/10.1371/journal.pone.0039731] [PMID: 22761880]

[24]   Damoiseaux JS, Beckmann CF, Arigita EJS, *et al.* Reduced resting-state brain activity in the "default network" in normal aging. Cereb Cortex 2008; 18(8): 1856-64.
[http://dx.doi.org/10.1093/cercor/bhm207] [PMID: 18063564]

[25]   Jones DT, Machulda MM, Vemuri P, *et al.* Age-related changes in the default mode network are more advanced in Alzheimer disease. Neurology 2011; 77(16): 1524-31.
[http://dx.doi.org/10.1212/WNL.0b013e318233b33d] [PMID: 21975202]

[26]   Jones DT, Knopman DS, Gunter JL, *et al.* Cascading network failure across the Alzheimer's disease spectrum. Brain 2016; 139(Pt 2): 547-62.
[http://dx.doi.org/10.1093/brain/awv338] [PMID: 26586695]

[27]   Zhou J, Gennatas ED, Kramer JH, Miller BL, Seeley WW. Predicting regional neurodegeneration from the healthy brain functional connectome. Neuron 2012; 73(6): 1216-27.
[http://dx.doi.org/10.1016/j.neuron.2012.03.004] [PMID: 22445348]

[28]   Jack CR Jr, Knopman DS, Jagust WJ, *et al.* Tracking pathophysiological processes in Alzheimer's disease: an updated hypothetical model of dynamic biomarkers. Lancet Neurol 2013; 12(2): 207-16.
[http://dx.doi.org/10.1016/S1474-4422(12)70291-0] [PMID: 23332364]

[29]   Petersen RC. Mild Cognitive Impairment. Continuum. Minneapolis, Minn 2016; 22: pp. (2 Dementia)404-18.

[30]   López-Sanz D, Bruña R, Garcés P, *et al.* Functional Connectivity Disruption in Subjective Cognitive Decline and Mild Cognitive Impairment: A Common Pattern of Alterations. Front Aging Neurosci 2017; 9(April): 109.
[http://dx.doi.org/10.3389/fnagi.2017.00109] [PMID: 28484387]

[31]   Garcés P, Angel Pineda-Pardo J, Canuet L, *et al.* The Default Mode Network is functionally and structurally disrupted in amnestic mild cognitive impairment - a bimodal MEG-DTI study. Neuroimage Clin 2014; 6: 214-21.
[http://dx.doi.org/10.1016/j.nicl.2014.09.004] [PMID: 25379433]

[32]   Canuet L, Pusil S, López ME, *et al.* Network Disruption and Cerebrospinal Fluid Amyloid-Beta and Phospho-Tau Levels in Mild Cognitive Impairment. J Neurosci 2015; 35(28): 10325-30.
[http://dx.doi.org/10.1523/JNEUROSCI.0704-15.2015] [PMID: 26180207]

[33]   López ME, Engels MMA, van Straaten ECW, *et al.* MEG Beamformer-Based Reconstructions of Functional Networks in Mild Cognitive Impairment. Front Aging Neurosci 2017; 9: 107.
[http://dx.doi.org/10.3389/fnagi.2017.00107] [PMID: 28487647]

[34]   Jiang ZY, Zheng LL. Inter- and intra-hemispheric EEG coherence in patients with mild cognitive impairment at rest and during working memory task. J Zhejiang Univ Sci B 2006; 7(5): 357-64.
[http://dx.doi.org/10.1631/jzus.2006.B0357] [PMID: 16615165]

[35]   Zheng LL, Jiang ZY, Yu EY. Alpha spectral power and coherence in the patients with mild cognitive impairment during a three-level working memory task. J Zhejiang Univ Sci B 2007; 8(8): 584-92.
[http://dx.doi.org/10.1631/jzus.2007.B0584] [PMID: 17657862]

[36]   Moretti D V, Miniussi C, Frisoni GB, *et al.* Hippocampal atrophy and EEG markers in subjects with mild cognitive impairment. Clinical neurophysiology : official journal of the International Federation of Clinical Neurophysiology 2007; 118: 2716-9.
[http://dx.doi.org/10.1016/j.clinph.2007.09.059]

[37]   Gómez C, Stam CJ, Hornero R, Fernández A, Maestú F. Disturbed beta band functional connectivity in patients with mild cognitive impairment: an MEG study. IEEE Trans Biomed Eng 2009; 56(6): 1683-90.
[http://dx.doi.org/10.1109/TBME.2009.2018454] [PMID: 19362905]

[38]   López ME, Bruña R, Aurtenetxe S, *et al.* Alpha-band hypersynchronization in progressive mild cognitive impairment: a magnetoencephalography study. J Neurosci 2014; 34(44): 14551-9.
[http://dx.doi.org/10.1523/JNEUROSCI.0964-14.2014] [PMID: 25355209]

[39]   Bajo R, Maestú F, Nevado A, *et al.* Functional connectivity in mild cognitive impairment during a memory task: implications for the disconnection hypothesis. J Alzheimers Dis 2010; 22(1): 183-93.
[http://dx.doi.org/10.3233/JAD-2010-100177] [PMID: 20847450]

[40]   Bajo R, Castellanos NP, Cuesta P, *et al.* Differential patterns of connectivity in progressive mild cognitive impairment. Brain Connect 2012; 2(1): 21-4.
[http://dx.doi.org/10.1089/brain.2011.0069] [PMID: 22458376]

[41]   Rémy F, Mirrashed F, Campbell B, Richter W. Mental calculation impairment in Alzheimer's disease: a functional magnetic resonance imaging study. Neurosci Lett 2004; 358(1): 25-8.
[http://dx.doi.org/10.1016/j.neulet.2003.12.122] [PMID: 15016426]

[42]   López ME, Garcés P, Cuesta P, *et al.* Synchronization during an Internally Directed Cognitive State in healthy aging and Mild Cognitive Impairment. A MEG study AGE (Dordr) 2014 Mar 23; IF: 4.084.

[43]   Buldú JM, Bajo R, Maestú F, *et al.* Reorganization of functional networks in mild cognitive impairment. PLoS One 2011; 6(5): e19584.
[http://dx.doi.org/10.1371/journal.pone.0019584] [PMID: 21625430]

[44]   Cirrito JR, Kang J-E, Lee J, *et al.* Endocytosis is required for synaptic activity-dependent release of amyloid-beta *in vivo.* Neuron 2008; 58(1): 42-51.
[http://dx.doi.org/10.1016/j.neuron.2008.02.003] [PMID: 18400162]

[45]   Garcia-Marin V, Blazquez-Llorca L, Rodriguez JR, *et al.* Diminished perisomatic GABAergic terminals on cortical neurons adjacent to amyloid plaques. Front Neuroanat 2009; 3: 28.
[http://dx.doi.org/10.3389/neuro.05.028.2009] [PMID: 19949482]

[46]   Garcés P, Vicente R, Wibral M, *et al.* Brain-wide slowing of spontaneous alpha rhythms in mild cognitive impairment. Front Aging Neurosci 2013; 5: 100.
[http://dx.doi.org/10.3389/fnagi.2013.00100] [PMID: 24409145]

[47]   Petersen RC. Mild cognitive impairment as a diagnostic entity. J Intern Med 2004; 256(3): 183-94.
[http://dx.doi.org/10.1111/j.1365-2796.2004.01388.x] [PMID: 15324362]

[48]   Winblad B, Palmer K, Kivipelto M, *et al.* Mild cognitive impairment--beyond controversies, towards a consensus: report of the International Working Group on Mild Cognitive Impairment. J Intern Med 2004; 256(3): 240-6.
[http://dx.doi.org/10.1111/j.1365-2796.2004.01380.x] [PMID: 15324367]

[49]   López ME, Cuesta P, Garcés P, *et al.* MEG spectral analysis in subtypes of Mild Cognitive Impairment. AGE 2014 (Dordr) 2014 Jun; 36(3): 9624.
[http://dx.doi.org/10.1007/s11357-014-9624-5]

[50]   Fernández A, Turrero A, Zuluaga P, *et al.* MEG delta mapping along the healthy aging-Alzheimer's disease continuum: diagnostic implications. J Alzheimers Dis 2013; 35(3): 495-507.
[http://dx.doi.org/10.3233/JAD-121912] [PMID: 23478303]

[51]   López ME, Turrero A, Cuesta P, *et al.* Searching for Primary Predictors of Conversion from Mild Cognitive Impairment to Alzheimer's Disease: A Multivariate Follow-Up Study. J Alzheimers Dis 2016; 52(1): 133-43.
[http://dx.doi.org/10.3233/JAD-151034] [PMID: 27060953]

[52]   Jessen F, Amariglio RE, van Boxtel M, *et al.* A conceptual framework for research on subjective cognitive decline in preclinical Alzheimer's disease. Alzheimers Dement 2014; 10(6): 844-52.
[http://dx.doi.org/10.1016/j.jalz.2014.01.001] [PMID: 24798886]

[53]   Wolfsgruber S, Kleineidam L, Wagner M, *et al.* Differential Risk of Incident Alzheimer's Disease Dementia in Stable Versus Unstable Patterns of Subjective Cognitive Decline. J Alzheimers Dis 2016; 54(3): 1135-46.
[http://dx.doi.org/10.3233/JAD-160407] [PMID: 27567852]

[54]   López-Sanz D, Bruña R, Garcés P, *et al.* Alpha band disruption in the AD-continuum starts in the Subjective Cognitive Decline stage: a MEG study. Sci Rep 2016; 6: 37685.
[http://dx.doi.org/10.1038/srep37685] [PMID: 27883082]

[55]   Visser PJ, Verhey F, Knol DL, *et al.* Prevalence and prognostic value of CSF markers of Alzheimer's disease pathology in patients with subjective cognitive impairment or mild cognitive impairment in the DESCRIPA study: a prospective cohort study. Lancet Neurol 2009; 8(7): 619-27.
[http://dx.doi.org/10.1016/S1474-4422(09)70139-5] [PMID: 19523877]

[56]   López-Sanz D, Garcés P, Álvarez B, Delgado-Losada ML, López-Higes R, Maestú F. Network disruption in the preclinical stages of alzheimer's disease: From subjective cognitive decline to mild cognitive impairment. Int J Neural Syst 2017; 27(8): 1750041.
[http://dx.doi.org/10.1142/S0129065717500411] [PMID: 28958179]

[57]   Cho H, Yang DW, Shon YM, *et al.* Abnormal integrity of corticocortical tracts in mild cognitive impairment: a diffusion tensor imaging study. J Korean Med Sci 2008; 23(3): 477-83.
[http://dx.doi.org/10.3346/jkms.2008.23.3.477] [PMID: 18583886]

[58]   Fonteijn HM, Norris DG, Verstraten FA. Exploring the anatomical basis of effective connectivity models with DTI-based fiber tractography. Int J Biomed Imaging 2008; 2008: 423192.
[http://dx.doi.org/10.1155/2008/423192] [PMID: 18483617]

[59]   Fellgiebel A, Wille P, Müller MJ, *et al.* Ultrastructural hippocampal and white matter alterations in mild cognitive impairment: a diffusion tensor imaging study. Dement Geriatr Cogn Disord 2004; 18(1): 101-8.
[http://dx.doi.org/10.1159/000077817] [PMID: 15087585]

[60]   Maggipinto T, Bellotti R, Amoroso N, *et al.* DTI measurements for Alzheimer's classification. Phys Med Biol 2017; 62(6): 2361-75.
[http://dx.doi.org/10.1088/1361-6560/aa5dbe] [PMID: 28234631]

[61]   Marcos Dolado A, Garcia Azorin D, Yus Fuertes M, *et al.* Conectividad cerebral y riesgo de evolución a Enfermedad de Alzheimer. Proceedings of the LXVIII Annual Meeting of the Sociedad Española de Neurología Ediciones SEN.

CHAPTER 3

Pain and Dementia

Enrique Arriola Manchola[1,*] and **Javier Alaba Trueba**[2]

[1] *Memory and Alzheimer Unit, Matiá Foundation, San Sebastián, Spain;*

[2] *Member of Dementia Group of the Spanish Society of Geriatrics and Gerontology (SEGG)*

Abstract: Pain assessment in the different stages of Alzheimer's disease can become complex, especially in the final stages of the disease due to the inability of patients to express the different characteristics of the pain, so it is necessary to use observational scales to detect pain "equivalents".

Keywords: Aging, Assessment, Behavior, Pain, Sementia.

INTRODUCTION

Population aging is creating new needs of care and this new reality is going to modify medical care, as well as the social and economic policies of the developed countries.

Following the Spanish Census of 2003, the aging index is 17% (people aged 65 or older). According to population projections, it is estimated that in 2050 this percentage will reach 35%. Spain is, after Japan, the second most aged country in the world. The age bracket of people aged older than 80 is expected to grow continuously, and could reach 4% to 11%, causing the "aging of elderly people" effect [1, 2].

It is estimated that about 35 million people worldwide have dementia. Its incidence is greater than 5% in people aged 65 and 50% in those over age 90 [3]. Age constitutes a risk factor for pain and dementia. Dementia has a great influence on the expression of pain, making its detection more difficult.

Pain is a complex phenomenon derived from a sensory stimulus or neurological injury and modified by the individual's memory, its expectations and emotions. Pain has different components (sensitive, affective, cognitive, autonomic, *etc.*). In

---

* **Corresponding author Enrique Arriola Manchola:** Memory and Alzheimer Unit, Matiá Foundation, San Sebastián, Spain; Tel: +34 943 317100; Fax: 943 2155 33; E-mail: enrique.arriola@matiafundazioa.net

Blas Gil-Extremera (Ed.)

the absence of biological markers, the communication skills of the patient are considered the standard test for diagnosis and pain quantification [4]. Pain should be considered as a geriatric syndrome, causing functional impairment of multifactorial etiology and whose identification depends on multidisciplinary assessment.

In general, we can say that aged people are more vulnerable to pain because they have decreased physiological reserves due to the aging process itself as well as chronic and incurable health problems (diabetes, hypertension, osteoporosis, osteoarthritis and heart failure...); they also have a diminished social network caused by personal losses which directly affects their care and psychological support. These circumstances could contribute to a possible reduction in pain threshold.

Malignant pain is more common with aging, since the presence of neoplasms increases with age. Thus, 60% of all neoplasms and 70% of all deaths caused by cancer develop in people older than 65 years.

Comorbidity with pain is a usual process accompanying the most frequent dementia processes (vascular dementia and Alzheimer's disease) as shown in several epidemiological studies [5, 6]; also elderly people have a high prevalence of painful diseases and geriatric syndromes that present with pain (immobility, pressure ulcers, fecal impaction, *etc.*). The prevalence of nociceptive pain in elderly people is of 25-50% [7] in the community, reaching 49-83% in gerontology centers [8, 9]. In 40% of cases, an adequate control of pain can not be reached. On the other hand, it is known that in these segments of the population, the use of opioids is less frequent [10, 11].

In our study [12] carried out on elderly institutionalized subjects, we studied 187 residents with a mean age of 84 years (74% women); 40% of them had severe dependence, and the prevalence of dementia was found in 64% of the residents. The prevalence of pain was 61%, mainly nociceptive/somatic pain related to osteoarticular pathologies; in 64% of the patients the pain was present everyday, and in 29% the pain was severe. There was a correlation between the presence of pain and the functional ability and the level of anxiety. 22% of patients with dementia presented scores > 4 according to the PAINAD scale showing a correlation between the presence of pain and the functional capacity, emotional state and behavior; a low correlation (r: 0.24) was found between behavioral disorders and the presence of pain. However, pain is usually present as confusion, behavioral disorders, decreased mobility and antalgic positions that finally cause primary caregiver burden [13].

To conduct a proper assessment of pain in patients with communication problems, it is essential to have appropriate information provided by the usual formal (professionals) and informal (family) caregivers. It must be pointed out that 23% of the residents studied had a creatinine clearance < 30 ml/min, considering the risks of toxicity of renal elimination such as opioids, so the adequate management of these drugs requires a dose reduction or a longer dosage interval in order to improve tolerance levels.

The evolution of the prevalence of institutionalized patients with dementia over time in Guipúzcoa is as follows: 1995 (26%), 2000 (42%), 2006 (56%) 2007 (60%), 2011 (70%). Today the user profile in a Gerontology Center is: female, widow, older than 84 years and with severe cognitive and functional decline (Stage 6 in the FAST scale) and with a life expectancy between 0 and 2 years. Nursing homes for dementia patients are at risk of becoming huge palliative care units. In this respect, we should bear in mind the short life expectancy of these patients (3-6 years) for an effective plan control [14 - 16].

Acute and chronic pain is an underestimated symptom and is undertreated in elderly patients, in general, and in dementia subjects in particular [17, 18]. Changes caused by aging with respect to pain perception are clinically insignificant [19], however, the use of opioids decreases with aging [20].

One of the factors influencing the underuse of therapeutic resources comes to find the medications due to the patient who assumes, that caused by these changes are inherent to age, and do not seek the fear of disturbing aspects and discomfort additional tests; family and some healthcare professionals also perceive these changes as typical of aging.

Sensory (vision and hearing) and communication problems make an adequate assessment of pain more difficult; also the fear of adverse drugs reactions limits the use of drugs suitable for the adequate pain control.

The consequences of untreated pain include depression, insomnia, and cardiovascular (due to adrenergic overstimulation) and neuroendocrine morbidity, reduced cognitive function, reduction of functional skills, socialization, social isolation, increased costs due to over-utilization of the health services, socially inappropriate behavior, resistance to care, delusions, reduced wandering [21], physical inactivity [22] and [23] sleep disorders.

SOME REAL-WORLD OBSERVATIONS

1. We found a lower use of analgesics in patients with dementia in the postoperative period (1/3 less morphine) [24] and in patients with significant daily pain [25] and that they complaining less about pain.

2. A decrease in affective components of pain is found in patients with frontotemporal dementia whereas subjects with vascular dementia showed an increase in affective pain experience [26].

3. AD patients reported less pain because the neuropathological lesions of AD patients in the locus coeruleus, periaqueductal gray matter, thalamus, insula, amygdala and hypothalamus alter all the components of pain perception: emotional, cognitive component and memory formation [26]. These lesions also affect pain threshold and autonomic and vegetative response [27].

4. Patients do not show either vegetative or neuroendocrine changes until more intense painful stimuli [28] are applied. According to the Acute *versus* Chronic Pain Questionnaire (ACPQ), patients with AD perceive much more acute pain than chronic pain [29]. Neuropathological involvement in AD seems to preserve, at least in the initial stages, the lateral pain system, which is responsible for the sensory aspects of pain and other threshold which is also altered. The medial system responsible for the other painful components (emotional, affective, cognitive, autonomic) is most affected, which means a greater tolerance to chronic pain.

5. It was found that patients with cognitive impairment and preserved verbal ability [17] are able to describe the pain when it is present, but are unable to describe it 24 hours later, *i.e.* it is necessary to measure the pain more frequently to detect it.

6. We must bear in mind that communication problems [30] occur in up to one-third of patients; difficulties increase as cognitive impairment advances, causing that these patients are sometimes undertreated.

7. In a retrospective and comparative study of patients with cancer and patients with dementia [31], the symptoms most commonly reported in the last year of life were mental confusion (83%), urinary incontinence (72%), pain (64%), depressive mood (61%), constipation (59%) and loss of appetite (57%). Patients with dementia received the visit of their general practitioners less often than cancer patients. The respondents rated the assistance of these professionals less favorably when the severity of the symptoms identified seemed to indicate healthcare needs similar in both groups.

8. It has been established that patients with dementia and hip fracture receive one third the morphine of controls and that 44% of controls report severe or very severe pain in the preoperative period and 42% during postoperative recovery [32].

9. A total of 523 patients older than 75 were interviewed in a study carried out by Mantyselka [25], where the prevalence rates of any pain, any daily pain, daily pain interfering with routine activity, and pain that requires resting were measured in patients with dementia (43%, 23%, 19% and 4%) *versus* patients without dementia (69%, 40%, 36% and 13%), respectively. Patients with

dementia took less analgesics (33%) than those without dementia (47%).
10. AD patients reported more pain in the early stages of the disease than those in a more advanced stage of the disease.

These comments, which need to be taken into account in order to assess pain in patients with dementia, are historically related with our appreciation of a lower use of analgesics in these patients in circumstances that are medically similar. Do patients with dementia feel less pain or are we not adequately measuring with a sensitive tool the presence and intensity of it?

PAIN ASSESSMENT IN PATIENTS WITH DEMENTIA

Morphological and functional changes that occur in the body as we age are numerous, as well as the neuropathological changes caused by the different dementia syndromes which modify the different processing mechanisms and pain regulation [33].

When studying the phenomenon of pain in patients with dementia, different types of pain must be differentiated (nociceptive, neuropathic, mixed), as well as its temporality (acute, subacute, chronic, persistent) and etiology of dementia (the different nature and location of the lesions affect the processing of pain). In addition, pain has cognitive, affective, autonomic and behavioral components, taking into consideration the level of disability they generate.Patients with vascular dementia have increased emotional pain, since white matter lesions increase the sensitivity by differentiation, being related to the presence of central pain [34].

Frontotemporal dementia patients show a reduction of processing and the emotional component of pain, presenting a greater tolerance to it [35].

In dementia with Lewy bodies, there is a reduction of the perception of pain and suffering, being similar to the of the EA white matter lesions, however the fundamental alteration occurs in the perisylvian area [36].

Assessing pain in older persons with dementia, especially in advanced stages, is a challenge. Although there is pain perception in cognitive impairment, often it is not reported because many of these people have lost the verbal skills to express it or because sometimes the nature of your condition may be blocking their ability to identify it. Also, for caregivers and professionals, identifying pain in people with dementia is quite complex because of, among other things, inadequate training or training to identify it [37] (see Table **1**).

Table 1. Barriers and strategies for a successful estimation of the pain.

Barriers	Strategies to Overcome the Barriers
Lacking in recognition. Insufficient formation and / or training misdiagnosis or late diagnosis. Not use of assessment tools Stoic attitudes.	To meet the person To recognize the diversity / intuitive perception Education and training Adequate tools

When performing auto reports of pain, compared to those prepared by professional caregivers, both physicians and nurses tend to underestimate the intensity of the pain of the patient [38]. On the other hand, family caregivers are more likely to overestimate the intensity of pain [39]. In the early stages of dementia, one can be safely use Visual Scales Analog [40]. In the intermediate stages the loss of abstract reasoning, the concepts in the scales may not be adequately understood [41]. In advanced stage, the patients don't understand or are unable to understand even simple scales [42] (see Table **2**).

Table 2. Measurement of pain in the cognitive impairment.

- In the early stages of dementia, analog visual scales can be useful [28]. - In the intermediate stages of dementia, the loss of abstract reasoning may lead to the possible misunderstanding of the concepts used in the scales [29]. - In advance stage of the disease, patients are not able to understand the most simple scales [17].

The need to use observational scales to assess pain in patients with advanced dementia can be problematic since expressions of pain are less obvious than people those given by without dementia and can be confounded issues of social rejection, aggression, confusion, behavioral changes, which are not typical of pain manifestations. Recent studies suggest that nurses, caregivers, family members and assistants can recognize the presence, but not the intensity, of pain in patients who are that is directly compared with those who can cognitively disabled [43 - 47].

Direct observation of patient behavior and besides those equivalent is verbalize their perceptions is necessary to be able to estimate the pain of patients with verbal disability / alternative ways to gauge the level of pain are needed to determine the degree of pain in this population. The knowledge of this information led to the American Society of Geriatrics [48] to insist on improving the evaluation of pain in patients with cognitive impairment. Thus, in its clinical guidelines, they identify six types of pain manifestation/equivalent (see Table **3**).

Table 3. Behavioral indicators of pain in elderly persons with dementia, according to the American Geriatrics Society (AGS).

1. Facial expressions: wrinkled forehead, face of sadness or fear, grimacing, closed or tightened eyes, constant blinking, distorted expressions.
2. Verbalizations, vocalizations: Sighing, moaning, groaning, grunting, chanting, calling out, noisy breathing, constantly asking for help, Verbally abusive language.
3. Body movements: rigidity, tense body posture, guarding attitude, fidgeting
Increased pacing, rocking, restriction in movements, mobility changes
4. Changes in interpersonal interactions: aggressivity, combative attitude, resisting care, social isolation, inappropriate reactions.
5. Changes in routines: refusing food, appetite change; increased rest periods,
Sleep, rest pattern changes, sudden cessation of common routines, increased wandering.
6. Mental status changes: crying or tears, increased confusion, irritability or distress

However there are two comprehensive reviews of scales of pain assessment in insane that partially included the recommended items, and its psychometrics have just been recommended [44, 49 - 51]: DS-DAT (DISCOMFORT IN DEMENTIA OF THE ALZHEIMER'S TYPE) [52] could be excluded because the concept of discomfort differs from pain but considers that it should be included and would be the first choice for many), PACSLAC (PAIN ASSESSMENT CHECKLIST FOR SENIORS WITH LIMITED ABILITY TO COMMUNICATE) [53] and the DOLOPLUS2 [54] and PAINAD (PAIN ASSESSMENT IN ADVANCED DEMENTIA SCALE) [55].

For this, we must include the number of items in the assessment that includes each tool of AGS and the quality of studies used to assess pain (see Tables **4** and **5**).

Table 4. Comparison of scales in relation to AGS indicators.

Scales	DS-DAT	DOLOPLUS	PACSLAC	PAINAD
Facial expression		X	X	X
Vocalization	X	X	X	X
Body movements	X	X	X	X
Changes in interpersonal interactions		X	X	
Changes in routines		X		
Mental status changes	X		X	

Table 5. Pain assessment scales.

	Construct	Subjects	Administration and Rating	Reliability	Validity	Total
ABBEY	1	1	1	1	1	5
PACSLAC	2	2	2	2	2	10
DS-DAT	2	2	1	2	2	9
NOPPAIN	2	2	2	2	2	10
PAINAD	2	3	3	3	2	13

3 = strong evidences; 2 = need for further studies; 1 = poor evidences; 0 = no evidences.

There are other instruments of great interest such as NOPPAIN (Non-Communicative Patient´s Pain Assessment Instrument) [56] that can be administered by auxiliary staff. The PAINAD designed by Volicer [55] that we understand also can help us assess the existence and intensity of pain, which will result in better clinical practice. In a cross-sectional study to search for predictors of situations that cause pain in these patients it was proved that physical constraint, dependence for the bathroom and the need for assistance for transfers were the moments in which the PAINAD yielded higher scores [57].

Slow but progressive models of quality assurance which includes indicators of pain control in vulnerable elders [58] are being incorporated (see Table **6**).

Table 6. Quality indicators for pain management in vulnerable elders.

Indicators 1 & 2: Screening for chronic pain at new visit of patients Indicator 3: History and physical examination for pain Indicator 4: Risks assessment by using nonsteroidal anti-Inflammatory drugs Indicator 5: Prevention of constipation in patients using opioids Indicator 6: Treatment of pain Indicator 7: Reassessment of pain control

Nurses observed that the pain assessment in these patients produced an increased use of analgesics with the consequent reduction of pain; in relation to nursing staff, it produced a reduction of stress and "burnout" [59]. The high prevalence of comorbidity in activity (malnutrition, incontinence, ulcers by pressure, delirium, depression, diabetes, cardio and cerebrovascular, respiratory problems) and the frequency of pain complicate tremendously the assistance of these patients, therefore the physicians working in this environment must be particularly attentive and vigilant (see Table **7**) to detect the existence and treatment of pain in patients with advanced dementia [60], especially during bathing, physical containment and assisted transfers [57].

Table 7. Distressing pathologies (RED FLAGS) to be excluded as a matter of priority in old people with pain.

1.- Herpes Zoster infection
2.- Temporal arteritis / polymyalgia rheumatica
3.- Traumatic injuries
4.- Nocturnal bone pain or rest pain indicative of malignancy, inflammation or infection.
5.- Limb ischemia

Assessment of pain is not easy, the scales that have been developed are multiple, and almost all of them are not validated in our population.Experts concluded that given the complexity of the assessment and interpretation of the DS-DAT, and the extension of the PACSLAC items, the PAINAD could be [61] the most practical scale. However, further knowledge and development of instruments are necessary to test more accurately pain in patients with advanced cognitive impairment [62].

If our goal as providers of health services is to provide comfort, "no pain" and reduce suffering of patients, we have the ethical duty to consider how we are going to measure these aspects in cognitively impaired patients [63]. That has been the reason for our validation of the PAINAD in the Spanish population with dementia [64] (see Table **8** and Annex **1**).

Table 8. PAINAD (Pain Assessment in Advanced Dementia).

	0	1	2	Score
Breathing independent of vocalization and verbalization of pain sensation	Normal	Occasional labored breathing Short periods of hyperventilation	Labored and noisy breathing Long periods of hyperventilation Cheyne-Stokes respiration.	
Negative vocalization/verbalization	None	Occasional groans, Low level of speech with disapproval.	Repeated and agitated calls. Loud level of groans, Crying	
Facial expression	Smiling or inexpressive	Sad, frightened, angry frown,	Grimaces of disapproval	
Body language	Relaxed	Tense, fidgeting, distressed pacing.	Rígid, clenched fists, Knees bent, pulling or pushing, physical aggressiveness	
Consolability	No need to console	Distracted or reassured with voice or touch	Unable to console, distract or reassure	
TOTAL				

PAIN AND BEHAVIORAL AND PSYCHOLOGICAL SYMPTOMS IN DEMENTIA (BPSD)

Behavioral disorders occur in all types of dementia and almost in 100% of cases during their progression time course. The BPSD can result from many causes (see Table **9**).

Table 9. Possible causes of behavioral disorders.

• Discomfort
• Unmet needs for physical care
• Conflicts with persons and environment (agitation imbalances)
• Reactions to stress
• Unclear/idiopathic cause
• An "equivalent" of pain

It was Husebo *et al.* [65] who carried out the first systematic review trying to associate pain with behavioral disorders in patients with dementia; they found that dementia improved with analgesic treatment in PubMed and the Cochrane database since 1992-2010, appreciating that the results were inconsistent and that randomized controlled studies were needed. The same authors carried out a study [66] demonstrating that effective control of pain, reduced agitation in institutionalized elderly with moderate - severe dementia. The finding merited an editorial in the British Medical Journal [67] and the assessment of pain or discomfort is already in the guidelines of excellence [68]. Subsequent works have directly linked pain with more delirium symptoms, lower physical function and increased risk of mortality [69, 70]. Physical inactivity in patients with dementia may be confused with apathy and be caused by pain; this may also occur in people without dementia. Pain caused by osteoarthritis of the hip, arthritis and back pain reduce physical activity; physical inactivity causes pain due to immobility. In older people with dementia pain may cause physical inactivity and vice versa [22], and this aspect should be considered. Likewise, also sleep problems have been associated with pain; these patients also present more frequently insomnia induction and restless sleep [23]

PAIN TREATMENT IN OLD PEOPLE WITH DEMENTIA

In the pharmacological treatment of pain, we must take into account the physiological changes that cause aging. These pharmacokinetics impact and the use of pharmacodynamics of drugs, comorbidity, drug interactions and the non-use of placebos for pain. The "expectation" placebo component disappears with the involvement of the frontal areas (executive function) in patients with Alzheimer's disease and especially in patients with dementia affecting the frontal lobe [71].

CONCLUSIONS

In patients with advanced dementia:

1. We must explore the existence of pain in a systematic way including pain caused by health problems or injury.
2. We must have tools that help us to measure the presence of pain and its intensity.
3. The existence of pain must be considered as a causative or contributory factor for disorders of behavior, sleep, or mobility, including therapeutic trial for pain prior to the use of psychotropic drugs.

ANNEX 1

Definitions of items

Breathing

1. Normal breathing: characterized by effortless, quiet, and rhythmic respirations.
2. Occasional labored breathing: characterized by episodic bursts of harsh, difficult or wearing respirations.
3. Short period of hyperventilation: characterized by intervals of rapid, deep breaths lasting a short period of time.
4. Noisy labored breathing: characterized by negative sounding respirations on inspiration or expiration. They may be loud, gurgling, or wheezing. They appear strenuous or wearing.
5. Long periods of hyperventilation: characterized by an excessive rate and depth of respirations lasting a considerable time.
6. Cheyne-Stokes respirations: characterized by rhythmic waxing and waning of breathing from very deep to shallow respirations with periods of apnea (cessation of breathing).

Negative Verbalization/Vocalization

1. None: characterized by speech or vocalization with neutral or pleasant quality.
2. Occasional groans: characterized by mournful or murmuring sounds, wails or laments. Groaning is characterized by inarticulate involuntary sounds louder than usual, often with abrupt beginning and ending.
3. Murmmur with a negative or disapproving quality: characterized by muttering, mumbling, whining, grumbling, or swearing in a low volume with a complaining, sarcastic tone.

4. Repeated agitated calls: characterized by phrases or words being used over and over in a tone suggesting anxiety, or distress.
5. Loud groaning: characterized by murmuring sounds, wails or laments with a louder than usual volume. Loud groans: characterized inarticulate involuntary sounds louder than usual and often with abrupt beginning and ending.
6. Crying: characterized by an utterance of emotion accompanied by tears. There may be sobbing or quiet weeping.

Facial Expression

1. Smiling: characterized by upturned corners of the mouth, brightening of the eyes and a look of pleasure Inexpressive: a neutral, relaxed, or blank look.
2. Sad: characterized by an unhappy, lonesome, sorrowful, or dejected look. There may be tears in the eyes.
3. Frightened: characterized by a look of fear, alarm or heightened anxiety. Eyes wide open.
4. Angry frown: characterized by a downward turn of the corners of the mouth. Increased facial wrinkling in the forehead and around the mouth may appear.
5. Facial grimaces: characterized by a distorted, distressed look. The brow is more wrinkled as is the area around the mouth. Eyes may be squeezed shut.

Body Language

1. Relaxed: characterized by a calm, restful, mellow appearance. The person seems to be calm.
2. Tense: characterized by a strained and worried appearance. The jaw may be clenched (excluding any contracture).
3. Distressed pacing: characterized by activity that seems unsettled (unable to be still in a small space). There may be a fearful, worried, or disturbed element present. The rate may be faster or slower than normal.
4. Fidgeting: characterized by restless movement. The person fidgets with hands or squirms when in his seat, and might be hitching a chair across the room. Repetitive touching, rubbing body parts can also be observed.
5. Rigid; characterized by stiffening of the body. The arms and/or legs are tight and inflexible. The trunk may be straight and unyielding (excluding any contracture).
6. Clenched fists: characterized by tightly closed hands that may be opened and closed repeatedly.
7. Knees bent: characterized by flexing the legs up toward the chest. Overall altered appearance (excluding any contracture).
8. Opposition (pushing and pulling): characterized by active resistance and contrary to approach or care.
9. Physical aggression: characterized by hitting, kicking, grabbing, punching,

biting, or other forms of attack.

Consolability

1. No need to console: characterized by a sense of well being. The person seems to be happy.
2. Distracted or reassured by voice or touch: characterized by a disruption in the behavior when the person is spoken or touched. During the period of interaction, the person has no signs of discomfort.
3. Unable to console, distract or reassure: characterized by the inability to sooth the person or stop a behavior with words or actions.

ACKNOWLEDGEMENTS

Declared none

CONFLICT OF INTEREST

The authors confirm that this chapter content has no conflict of interest.

CONSENT FOR PUBLICATION

Not applicable.

REFERENCES

[1]   Abellán A. Indicadores demográficos. 2004.

[2]   de Trabajo M, Sociales A, Eds. Bases demográficas: estimación, características y perfiles de las personas en situación de dependencia.Libro Blanco Atención a las personas en situación de dependencia en España. Madrid: Ministerio de Trabajo y Asuntos Sociales 2005; pp. 19-92.

[3]   Klapwijk MS, Caljouw MA, van Soest-Poortvliet MC, van der Steen JT, Achterberg WP. Symptoms and treatment when death is expected in dementia patients in long-term care facilities. BMC Geriatr 2014; 14: 99.
        [http://dx.doi.org/10.1186/1471-2318-14-99] [PMID: 25181947]

[4]   Marin Carmona JM, Arriola Manchola E. Know Alzheimer. Manual de Consulta para Geriatras. Barcelona. Ed Profarmaco 2014; 2: 66-8.

[5]   Imfelda P, Brauchli Pernusa Y, Jickc S. Meiera Ch. Epidemiology, Co-Morbidities, and Medication Use of Patients with Alzheimer's Disease or Vascular Dementia in the UK. J Alzheimers Dis 2013; 35: 1-5.
        [PMID: 23364138]

[6]   Andersen F, Viitanen M, Halvorsen DS, Straume B, Engstad TA. Co-morbidity and drug treatment in Alzheimer's disease. A cross sectional study of participants in the dementia study in northern Norway. BMC Geriatr 2011; 11: 58.
        [http://dx.doi.org/10.1186/1471-2318-11-58] [PMID: 21970467]

[7]   Scherder E, Herr K, Pickering G, Gibson S, Benedetti F, Lautenbacher S. Pain in dementia. Pain 2009; 145(3): 276-8.
        [http://dx.doi.org/10.1016/j.pain.2009.04.007] [PMID: 19409705]

[8]   Kunz M, Mylius V, Scharmann S, Schepelman K, Lautenbacher S. Influence of dementia on multiple components of pain. Eur J Pain 2009; 13(3): 317-25.
[http://dx.doi.org/10.1016/j.ejpain.2008.05.001] [PMID: 18562225]

[9]   Ferrell BA. Pain evaluation and management in the nursing home. Ann Intern Med 1995; 123(9): 681-7.
[http://dx.doi.org/10.7326/0003-4819-123-9-199511010-00007] [PMID: 7574224]

[10]   Fries BE, Simon SE, Morris JN, Flodstrom C, Bookstein FL. Pain in U.S. nursing homes: validating a pain scale for the minimum data set. Gerontologist 2001; 41(2): 173-9.
[http://dx.doi.org/10.1093/geront/41.2.173] [PMID: 11327482]

[11]   Fox PL, Raina P, Jadad AR. Prevalence and treatment of pain in older adults in nursing homes and other long-term care institutions: a systematic review. CMAJ 1999; 160(3): 329-33.
[PMID: 10065074]

[12]   Álaba J, Arriola E. Prevalencia de dolor en pacientes geriátricos institucionalizados. Rev Soc Esp Dolor 2009; 16(6): 344-51.
[http://dx.doi.org/10.1016/S1134-8046(09)72542-X]

[13]   Benedetti F, Vighetti S, Ricco C, et al. Pain threshold and tolerance in Alzheimer's disease. Pain 1999; 80(1-2): 377-82.
[http://dx.doi.org/10.1016/S0304-3959(98)00228-0] [PMID: 10204751]

[14]   Brodaty H, Seeher K, Gibson L. Dementia time to death: a systematic literature review on survival time and years of life lost in people with dementia. Int Psychogeriatr 2012; 24(7): 1034-45.
[http://dx.doi.org/10.1017/S1041610211002924] [PMID: 22325331]

[15]   James BD, Leurgans SE, Hebert LE, Scherr PA, Yaffe K, Bennett DA. Contribution of Alzheimer disease to mortality in the United States. Neurology 2014; 82(12): 1045-50.
[http://dx.doi.org/10.1212/WNL.0000000000000240] [PMID: 24598707]

[16]   Wattmo C, Londos E, Minthon L. Risk factors that affect life expectancy in Alzheimer's disease: a 15-year follow-up. Dement Geriatr Cogn Disord 2014; 38(5-6): 286-99.
[http://dx.doi.org/10.1159/000362926] [PMID: 24992891]

[17]   Stein WM. Pain in the nursing home. Clin Geriatr Med 2001; 17(3): 575-594, viii.
[http://dx.doi.org/10.1016/S0749-0690(05)70098-7] [PMID: 11459722]

[18]   Feldt KS, Ryden M, Miles S. Treatment of pain in cognitively impaired with cognitively intact older patients with hip-fracture. JAGS 1998; pp. 1079-85.

[19]   Harkins SW. Geriatric pain. Pain perceptions in the old. Clin Geriatr Med 1996; 12(3): 435-59.
[http://dx.doi.org/10.1016/S0749-0690(18)30210-6] [PMID: 8853938]

[20]   Zyczkowska J, Szczerbińska K, Jantzi MR, Hirdes JP. Pain among the oldest old in community and institutional settings. Pain 2007; 129(1-2): 167-76.
[http://dx.doi.org/10.1016/j.pain.2006.12.009] [PMID: 17250966]

[21]   Tosato M, Lukas A, van der Roest HG, et al. Association of pain with behavioral and psychiatric symptoms among nursing home residents with cognitive impairment: results from the SHELTER study. Pain 2012; 153(2): 305-10.
[http://dx.doi.org/10.1016/j.pain.2011.10.007] [PMID: 22093815]

[22]   Plooij B, Scherder EJA, Eggermont LHP. Physical inactivity in aging and dementia: a review of its relationship to pain. J Clin Nurs 2012; 21(21-22): 3002-8.
[http://dx.doi.org/10.1111/j.1365-2702.2011.03856.x] [PMID: 22458668]

[23]   Chen Q, Hayman LL, Shmerling RH, Bean JF, Leveille SG, Leveille SG. Characteristics of chronic pain associated with sleep difficulty in older adults: the Maintenance of Balance, Independent Living, Intellect, and Zest in the Elderly (MOBILIZE) Boston study. J Am Geriatr Soc 2011; 59(8): 1385-92.
[http://dx.doi.org/10.1111/j.1532-5415.2011.03544.x] [PMID: 21806564]

[24]   Morrison RS, Siu AL. Survival in end-stage dementia following acute illness. JAMA 2000; 284(1): 47-52.
[http://dx.doi.org/10.1001/jama.284.1.47] [PMID: 10872012]

[25]   Mäntyselkä P, Hartikainen S, Louhivuori-Laako K, Sulkava R. Effects of dementia on perceived daily pain in home-dwelling elderly people: a population-based study. Age Ageing 2004; 33(5): 496-9.
[http://dx.doi.org/10.1093/ageing/afh165] [PMID: 15271639]

[26]   Scherder EJA, Sergeant JA, Swaab DF. Pain processing in dementia and its relation to neuropathology. Lancet Neurol 2003; 2(11): 677-86.
[http://dx.doi.org/10.1016/S1474-4422(03)00556-8] [PMID: 14572736]

[27]   Rainero I, Vighetti S, Bergamasco B, Pinessi L, Benedetti F. Autonomic responses and pain perception in Alzheimer's disease. Eur J Pain 2000; 4(3): 267-74.
[http://dx.doi.org/10.1053/eujp.2000.0185] [PMID: 10985870]

[28]   Burns A, Gallagley A, Byrne J. Delirium. J Neurol Neurosurg Psychiatry 2004; 75(3): 362-7.
[http://dx.doi.org/10.1136/jnnp.2003.023366] [PMID: 14966146]

[29]   Scherder EJ, Bouma A. Acute *versus* chronic pain experience in Alzheimer's disease. a new questionnaire. Dement Geriatr Cogn Disord 2000; 11(1): 11-6.
[http://dx.doi.org/10.1159/000017207] [PMID: 10629356]

[30]   Krulewitch H, London MR, Skakel VJ, Lundstedt GJ, Thomason H, Brummel-Smith K. Assessment of pain in cognitively impaired older adults: a comparison of pain assessment tools and their use by nonprofessional caregivers. J Am Geriatr Soc 2000; 48(12): 1607-11.
[http://dx.doi.org/10.1111/j.1532-5415.2000.tb03871.x] [PMID: 11129750]

[31]   McCarthy M, Addington-Hall J, Altmann D. The experience of dying with dementia: a retrospective study. Int J Geriatr Psychiatry 1997; 12(3): 404-9.
[http://dx.doi.org/10.1002/(SICI)1099-1166(199703)12:3<404::AID-GPS529>3.0.CO;2-2] [PMID: 9152728]

[32]   Morrison RS, Siu AL. A comparison of pain and its treatment in advanced dementia and cognitively intact patients with hip fracture. J Pain Symptom Manage 2000; 19(4): 240-8.
[http://dx.doi.org/10.1016/S0885-3924(00)00113-5] [PMID: 10799790]

[33]   Fine PG. Chronic pain management in older adults: special considerations. J Pain Symptom Manage 2009; 38(2) (Suppl.): S4-S14.
[http://dx.doi.org/10.1016/j.jpainsymman.2009.05.002] [PMID: 19671470]

[34]   Mori E. Impact of subcortical ischemic lesions on behavior and cognition. Ann N Y Acad Sci 2002; 977: 141-8.
[http://dx.doi.org/10.1111/j.1749-6632.2002.tb04809.x] [PMID: 12480744]

[35]   Bathgate D, Snowden JS, Varma A, Blackshaw A, Neary D. Behaviour in frontotemporal dementia, Alzheimer's disease and vascular dementia. Acta Neurol Scand 2001; 103(6): 367-78.
[http://dx.doi.org/10.1034/j.1600-0404.2001.2000236.x] [PMID: 11421849]

[36]   Burton EJ, Karas G, Paling SM, *et al.* Patterns of cerebral atrophy in dementia with Lewy bodies using voxel-based morphometry. Neuroimage 2002; 17(2): 618-30.
[http://dx.doi.org/10.1006/nimg.2002.1197] [PMID: 12377138]

[37]   McAuliffe L, O'Donnell M, Nay R. Successful pain assessment in older adults with dementia: barriers and strategies (review). Royal College of Nursing Australia Monograph. Australian Centre for Evidence Based Aged Care 2008.

[38]   Cohen-Mansfield J, Lipson S. Pain in cognitively impaired nursing home residents: how well are physicians diagnosing it? J Am Geriatr Soc 2002; 50(6): 1039-44.
[http://dx.doi.org/10.1046/j.1532-5415.2002.50258.x] [PMID: 12110063]

[39]   Madison JL, Wilkie DJ. Family members' perceptions of cancer pain. Comparisons with patient

sensory report and by patient psychologic status. Nurs Clin North Am 1995; 30(4): 625-45.
[PMID: 7501532]

[40]   Scherder EJ, Bouma A. Visual analogue scales for pain assessment in Alzheimer's disease. Gerontology 2000; 46(1): 47-53.
[http://dx.doi.org/10.1159/000022133] [PMID: 11111229]

[41]   Ferrell BA, Ferrell BR, Rivera L. Pain in cognitively impaired nursing home patients. J Pain Symptom Manage 1995; 10(8): 591-8.
[http://dx.doi.org/10.1016/0885-3924(95)00121-2] [PMID: 8594119]

[42]   Hurley AC, Volicer BJ, Hanrahan PA, Houde S, Volicer L. Assessment of discomfort in advanced Alzheimer patients. Res Nurs Health 1992; 15(5): 369-77.
[http://dx.doi.org/10.1002/nur.4770150506] [PMID: 1529121]

[43]   Cohen-Mansfield J, Creedon M. Nursing staff members' perceptions of pain indicators in persons with severe dementia. Clin J Pain 2002; 18(1): 64-73.
[http://dx.doi.org/10.1097/00002508-200201000-00010] [PMID: 11803305]

[44]   Fisher SE, Burgio LD, Thorn BE, *et al.* Pain assessment and management in cognitively impaired nursing home residents: association of certified nursing assistant pain report, Minimum Data Set pain report, and analgesic medication use. J Am Geriatr Soc 2002; 50(1): 152-6.
[http://dx.doi.org/10.1046/j.1532-5415.2002.50021.x] [PMID: 12028260]

[45]   Manfredi PL, Breuer B, Meier DE, Libow L. Pain assessment in elderly patients with severe dementia. J Pain Symptom Manage 2003; 25(1): 48-52.
[http://dx.doi.org/10.1016/S0885-3924(02)00530-4] [PMID: 12565188]

[46]   Mentes JC, Teer J, Cadogan MP. The pain experience of cognitively impaired nursing home residents: perceptions of family members and certified nursing assistants. Pain Manag Nurs 2004; 5(3): 118-25.
[http://dx.doi.org/10.1016/j.pmn.2004.01.001] [PMID: 15359223]

[47]   Shega JW, Hougham GW, Stocking CB, Cox-Hayley D, Sachs GA. Pain in community-dwelling persons with dementia: frequency, intensity, and congruence between patient and caregiver report. J Pain Symptom Manage 2004; 28(6): 585-92.
[http://dx.doi.org/10.1016/j.jpainsymman.2004.04.012] [PMID: 15589083]

[48]   The management of persistent pain in older persons. J Am Geriatr Soc 2002; 50(6) (Suppl.): S205-24.
[PMID: 12067390]

[49]   Herr K, Bjoro K, Decker S. Tools for assessment of pain in nonverbal older adults with dementia: a state-of-the-science review. J Pain Symptom Manage 2006; 31(2): 170-92.
[http://dx.doi.org/10.1016/j.jpainsymman.2005.07.001] [PMID: 16488350]

[50]   Zwakhalen SM, Hamers JP, Abu-Saad HH, Berger MP. Pain in elderly people with severe dementia: a systematic review of behavioural pain assessment tools. BMC Geriatr 2006; 6: 3.
[http://dx.doi.org/10.1186/1471-2318-6-3] [PMID: 16441889]

[51]   Malmstrom T, Tait R. Pain assessment and Management in older adults. 2010.
[http://dx.doi.org/10.1016/B978-0-12-374961-1.10024-7]

[52]   Hurley AC, Volicer BJ, Hanrahan PA, Houde S, Volicer L. Assessment of discomfort in advanced Alzheimer patients. Res Nurs Health 1992; 15(5): 369-77.
[http://dx.doi.org/10.1002/nur.4770150506] [PMID: 1529121]

[53]   Fuchs-Lacelle S, Hadjistavropoulos T. Development and preliminary validation of the pain assessment checklist for seniors with limited ability to communicate (PACSLAC). Pain Manag Nurs 2004; 5(1): 37-49.
[http://dx.doi.org/10.1016/j.pmn.2003.10.001] [PMID: 14999652]

[54]   Wary B, Doloplus C. Doloplus-2, une échelle pour évaluer la douleur. Soins Gerontol 1999; 19(19): 25-7.
[PMID: 10745928]

[55]   Warden V, Hurley AC, Volicer L. Development and psychometric evaluation of the Pain Assessment in Advanced Dementia (PAINAD) scale. J Am Med Dir Assoc 2003; 4(1): 9-15.
[http://dx.doi.org/10.1097/01.JAM.0000043422.31640.F7] [PMID: 12807591]

[56]   Snow AL, Weber JB, O'Malley KJ, *et al.* NOPPAIN: a nursing assistant-administered pain assessment instrument for use in dementia. Dement Geriatr Cogn Disord 2004; 17(3): 240-6.
[http://dx.doi.org/10.1159/000076446] [PMID: 14745230]

[57]   Lin P-C, Lin L-C, Shyu YI, Hua MS. Predictors of pain in nursing home residents with dementia: a cross-sectional study. J Clin Nurs 2011; 20(13-14): 1849-57.
[http://dx.doi.org/10.1111/j.1365-2702.2010.03695.x] [PMID: 21592246]

[58]   Chodosh J, Ferrell BA, Shekelle PG, Wenger NS. Quality indicators for pain management in vulnerable elders. Ann Intern Med 2001; 135(8 Pt 2): 731-5.
[http://dx.doi.org/10.7326/0003-4819-135-8_Part_2-200110161-00012] [PMID: 11601956]

[59]   Fuchs-Lacelle S, Hadjistavropoulos T, Lix L. Pain assessment as intervention: a study of older adults with severe dementia. Clin J Pain 2008; 24(8): 697-707.
[http://dx.doi.org/10.1097/AJP.0b013e318172625a] [PMID: 18806535]

[60]   Black BS, Finucane T, Baker A, *et al.* Health problems and correlates of pain in nursing home residents with advanced dementia. Alzheimer Dis Assoc Disord 2006; 20(4): 283-90.
[http://dx.doi.org/10.1097/01.wad.0000213854.04861.cc] [PMID: 17132974]

[61]   van Herk R, van Dijk, Baar FPM, Tibboel D, de Wit R. Observation scales for pain assessment in older adults with cognitive impairments or communication difficulties. Nursing Research _ January/February 2007; 56(1): 34-43.

[62]   Stolee P, Hillier LM, Esbaugh J, Bol N, McKellar L, Gauthier N. Instruments for the assessment of pain in older persons with cognitive impairment. J Am Geriatr Soc 2005; 53(2): 319-26.
[http://dx.doi.org/10.1111/j.1532-5415.2005.53121.x] [PMID: 15673359]

[63]   Arriola E, Alaba J. Comorbilidad medica en la enfermedad de Alzheimer evolucionada. En Aguera L, Bermejo F, Gil P. Monografía: Enfermedad de Alzheimer evolucionada. Med Clin (Barc) 2004; 5(6): 39-42.

[64]   García-Soler Á, Sánchez-Iglesias I, Buiza C, *et al.* Adaptación y validación de la versión española de la escala de evaluación de dolor en personas con demencia avanzada: PAINAD-Sp. Rev Esp Geriatr Gerontol 2014; 49(1): 10-4.
[http://dx.doi.org/10.1016/j.regg.2013.02.001] [PMID: 23746393]

[65]   Husebo BS, Ballard C, Aarsland D. Pain treatment of agitation in patients with dementia: a systematic review. Int J Geriatr Psychiatry 2011; 26(10): 1012-8.
[http://dx.doi.org/10.1002/gps.2649] [PMID: 21308784]

[66]   Husebo BS, Ballard C, Sandvik R, Nilsen OB, Aarsland D. Efficacy of treating pain to reduce behavioural disturbances in residents of nursing homes with dementia: cluster randomised clinical trial. BMJ 2011; 343: d4065.
[http://dx.doi.org/10.1136/bmj.d4065] [PMID: 21765198]

[67]   Rosenberg PB, Lyketsos CG. Treating agitation in dementia. BMJ 2011; 343: d3913.
[http://dx.doi.org/10.1136/bmj.d3913] [PMID: 21765197]

[68]   http://guidance.nice.org.uk/CG422006.

[69]   Kolanowski A, Mogle J, Fick DM, *et al.* Pain, delirium, and physical function in skilled nursing home patients with dementia. J Am Med Dir Assoc 2015; 16(1): 37-40.
[http://dx.doi.org/10.1016/j.jamda.2014.07.002] [PMID: 25239018]

[70]   Sampson EL, White N, Lord K, *et al.* Pain, agitation, and behavioural problems in people with dementia admitted to general hospital wards: a longitudinal cohort study. Pain 2015; 156(4): 675-83.
[http://dx.doi.org/10.1097/j.pain.0000000000000095] [PMID: 25790457]

[71]   Alaba J, Arriola E. Navarro, González MF, Buiza C, Hernández C, Zulaica A. Demencia y dolor. Rev Soc Esp Dolor 2011; 18(3): 176-86.

CHAPTER 4

Dysphagia in Alzheimer's Disease

J. García-Verdejo[1,*] and **L. Díaz-Rubia**[1]

[1] *Service of Internal Medicine, General Hospital, Motril, Spain*

[2] *Department of Radiology, "San Cecilio" Clinical Hospital, Granada, Spain*

Abstract: Patients with Alzheimer's disease may have dysphagia with greater frequency and severity in advanced stages of the disease. This can lead to complications such as dehydration, weight loss, malnutrition and aspiration pneumonia. Therefore, it is necessary to know the problem, identify it and treat it early. We can use postural modifications, changes in the volume and viscosity of food and ultimately the placement of a percutaneous endoscopic gastrostomy.

Keywords: Aspiration, Alzheimer's Disease, Dysphagia, Food, Nutrition, Swallowing.

INTRODUCTION

Swallowing is one of the basic functions of the organism. It is a complex neuromuscular process, involving more than 50 pairs of muscles and requiring a very precise coordination.

Dysphagia, or difficulty in swallowing, is classified according to place (oropharyngeal or esophageal) and mechanical or neurogenic. In the frequent elderly, an oropharyngeal dysphagia due to muscle and nervous system changes, that may lead to a global impoverishment of the motor response.

The prevalence of dysphagia in older individuals ranges from 7% to 22% and dramatically increases to 40% to 50% in older individuals who reside in long-term care facilities. Dysphagia can be a result of behavioral, sensory, or motor problems (or a combination of these) and is common in individuals with neurologic disease and dementia. Although there are few studies of the incidence and prevalence of dysphagia in individuals with dementia, it is estimated that 45% of institutionalized dementia patients have dysphagia. This means that this is a big problem and we do have to keep it in mind. The high prevalence of dysphagia in

---

* **Corresponding author Javier García-Verdejo:** Service of Internal Medicine, General Hospital of Motril, Granada, Spain; Tel: 685502076; Fax: 34 958038201; E-mail: verdejo@gmail.com

Blas Gil-Extremera (Ed.)

individuals with dementia likely is the result of age-related changes in sensory and motor function in addition to those produced by neuropathology [1].

Other conditions favoring dysphagia and aspiration in older people, such as the use of sedative medication (reduction of swallowing reflex) (Table **1**), decrease of saliva, loss of teeth and/or poor oral hygiene, are so frequent in the elderly that dysphagia has been postulated as a major geriatric syndrome, currently under-diagnosed.

Table 1. Drugs that can affect swallowing.

Drug	Effect
Antibiotics	Anorexia, Metallic taste, nausea
Anticholinergics	Xerostomia
Antipsychotic	Abnormal movements
Anxiolytic	Decreased attention
Bisphosphonates	Esophagitis, gastroesophageal reflux
Neuroleptics, sedatives, *etc.*	Decreased swallowing reflex
Toxic levels of drugs (*e.g.* digoxin)	Nausea

Alzheimer's disease (AD) is the prototype of cortical dementia. Dysphagia associated with this disease has been called pseudobulbar dysphagia and is a consequence of the involvement of the neocortex and the limbic system that impairs voluntary and stereotyped eating behaviors of the affected person [2].

In AD, the functional decline of the brain cortex region has been reported. Martin and Sessle [3] reviewed the association between the brain cortex and swallowing, and concluded that the brain cortex is in charge of the initiation and modification of swallowing and sensorimotor integration.

The destructuring of dietary behavior goes hand in hand with the severity of dementia, functional and cognitive loss, clinically affecting 45-50% of severe dementias of different etiologies. Its most important consequences are dehydration, weight loss, malnutrition and bronchoaspiration, with aspiration pneumonia being the main cause of death in these patients [4]. And the mortality caused by pneumonia in AD patients is particularly high when compared with subjects without dementia [5].

Typically, patients with dementia in their later stages are institutionalized. Facing dysphagia means facing the swallowing problem and its causes, the cognitive state, the nutritional status and its complications, including the end of life. This implies sensitization and knowledge of the problem, staff training, relationships with families and decision-making with variables as diverse as the scientific evidence or the personal beliefs of family members and caregivers [6].

DIAGNOSIS AND DETECTION

We know that the severity of AD is significantly associated with swallowing function [7]. So we need to detect dysphagia early and deal with it. Videoendoscopy (VE) and videofluorography (VF) are methods to assess oropharyngeal dysphagia and to examine swallowing function.

Those tests are difficult to undergo for AD patients because of the behavioral and psychological symptoms of dementia. Dysphagia can be managed using an approach based on a meal-time assessment and a thorough history [2].

Since the standard swallowing tests are often difficult to use for patients with dementia, we should use other methods to assess daily swallowing function in these patients.

One of the most important factors associated with dysphagia is "rinsing ability", so we need to analyze this in every patient with AD.

The diagnostic procedure for dysphagia starts from collecting patient information through history-taking, visual examination, palpation, *etc.* Patients suspected of having dysphagia proceed to the screening tests listed below. Based on test results, high-risk patients who are reasonably suspected of having dysphagia are screened, and if necessary, these patients proceed to more thorough examination such as video-fluorography or video-endoscopic examination of swallowing [8].

Simple Screening Tests

Below there are simple screening methods normally used to evaluate dysphagia.

Dry Swallowing

Humans repeat swallowing at certain intervals to get rid of saliva in the mouth, even when they do not eat. This dry swallowing is the basic movement used to eliminate saliva. Therefore, it is necessary to verify if the patient can swallow well before performing any other screening test.

Repetitive Saliva Swallowing Test (RSST)

This is a safe test to verify the patient's ability to swallow voluntarily. We measure the swallows in a certain period of time after giving the patient cold water [9].

Water Swallow Test

Water is difficult to swallow for patients with dysphagia, especially in patients with static dysphagia with poor food transport function due to cerebrovascular or neuromuscular disease. This test is intended to detect aspiration with high accuracy by having the patient swallow water. There are several methods using different quantities of water (30 mL, 3 mL). These methods may carry a risk of aspiration, especially using 30 ml. The one using 3 mL is called modified water swallowing test score (MWST).

It consists of pouring cold water into the mouth with a syringe, then the patient is given orders to swallow. We score those swallowing movements as in Table **2**. Dysphagia can be defined when the score is 3 or less. If the score is 4-5 the test is repeated and the lowest result is the definitive score [7].

Table 2. MWST scores.

Score 1	Inability to swallow with choking and/or breathing changes
Score 2	Swallowing occurred, but with breathing changes
Score 3	Swallowing occurred with no breathing changes, but with choking and/or wet hoarseness
Score 4	Swallowed successfully with no choking or wet hoarseness
Score 5	Furthermore to Score 4, additional deglutition (dry swallowing) occurred more than twice within 30 s

Colored Water Test

This test is used on tracheostomized patients. The patient is asked to swallow colored water to monitor any leakage from the tracheostomy incision.

Cervical Auscultation of Swallowing

Cervical auscultation during or after swallowing allows non-invasive assessment of aspiration or the presence of residual food in the pharynx. Changes in respiratory sound (mainly expiratory sound) and the presence of a respiratory murmur in the pharynx after swallowing are particularly important in the evaluation, such as wet sound, stenotic sound, whistling, gargles and liquid vibration [10].

Previous tests are not commonly used in patients with Alzheimer's disease, as their suitability has not been demonstrated. On the other hand, a test that has proved useful in the clinic is the Volume-Viscosity swallow test (V-VST), used to detect possible silent aspirations and based on observation of reactions of coughing, asphyxia and voice alteration.

Volume-Viscosity Swallow Test

The V-VST combines good psychometric properties, feasibility, a detailed and easy to perform protocol, an algorithm designed to protect patients' safety, enough end points to evaluate the safety and efficacy of swallowing, and a system to detect silent aspirations. The V-VST detects patients who need a diagnostic study (*e.g.* videofluoroscopy) or dietary modifications when the videofluoroscopy study is not possible.

In the hands of properly trained personnel, the diagnostic sensitivity of MECV-V for alterations the safety and efficacy of swallowing are the 88.1 and 89.8%, respectively. In addition to identifying to patients with dysphagia, the V-VST method identifies adequately to patients with safety of swallowing to which it is necessary to restrict liquid viscosity and provides data on the type of bolus (volume and viscosity) more suitable for each patient.

The risk of aspiration in patients with oropharyngeal dysphagia increases with decreasing viscosity of the fluids that are administered to the patient and by increasing the volume of the bolus. Therefore, a patient should not be exposed to a bolus of lower viscosity or higher volume (for the same viscosity) than that with which it has already shown signs of aspiration. The method uses three series of bowls of 5, 10 and 20 ml and of viscosity nectar, liquid and pudding; the test starts with viscosity medium and low volume to protect the patient and the exploration progresses through the administration of increasingly difficult boluses until the patient shows signs of aspiration. If the patient has oxygen desaturation or clinical signs of safety, the series is interrupted and passed to a series of higher viscosity [11].

Tests with Special Equipment Required

Measurement of Arterial Oxygen Saturation

We use a pulse oximeter to assess if there is a decrease in the partial pressure of O2 during the ingestion. If this occurs (with a decrease below 90% SpO_2), intake should be suspended to avoid aspiration risks. This does not directly detect an aspiration but it helps us to assess the respiratory state of the patient during meals [12].

Plain X-ray of the Neck

The patient is asked to swallow a small volume of contrast medium. By comparing plain X-ray images of the neck taken before and after the swallowing, conditions of laryngeal influx and the presence of aspiration or pharyngeal residue can be found. This method does not give us a dynamic monitoring of swallowing but it is easier and more accessible than videofluoroscopy since we don't need a special X-ray equipment.

Complementary Explorations

Pharyngoesophageal manometry and videofluoroscopy are complementary methods for the study of pathophysiology and the selection of the treatment of patients with oropharyngeal dysphagia and the alterations of opening of the upper esophageal sphincter. Videofluoroscopy (VFS) allows the identification of signs of safety and efficacy of swallowing, quantify the temporal events of the response oropharyngeal motor and establish the mechanisms of aspiration, measure hyoid movement and sphincter opening superior oesophageal pressure and the propulsive bolo, and manometry allows assessing the compliance of upper esophageal sphincter, hypopharyngeal pressure and mechanism of incomplete sphincter opening [13].

Videofluoroscopy

Videofluoroscopy (VFS) is a dynamic radiological technique consisting of obtaining a sequence in lateral and anteroposterior profile of the ingestion of different volumes and viscosities (liquid, nectar and pudding) of a water soluble contrast. At the moment this technique is considered the standard for the study of oropharyngeal dysphagia, since it allows to study the oropharyngeal motor response and to identify the videofluoroscopic signs. VFS allows the identification of 1/3 to 1/4 patients who are going to present clinically non-diagnosable silent aspirations and, therefore, will be at a very high risk of pneumonia. The objectives of videofluoroscopy are to evaluate the safety and efficacy of swallowing, to characterize swallowing alterations in terms of videofluoroscopic signs, to evaluate the efficacy of the treatments and to quantify the swallowing reflex [14].

Videofluoroscopic Signs of the Oral Phase

Main signs of alterations in the efficacy of the oral phase are the apraxia and decreased control and lingual propulsion of the bolus. Many patients have apraxia of swallowing (difficulty, delay or inability to start the oral phase) following a stroke, in AD and in patients with decrease in oral sensitivity. The alterations of the lingual control (inability to form the bolus) or propulsion cause an oral residue or in the vallecula when the alteration is from the base of the tongue. The main sign of the safety of the oral phase is the inadequacy of the of the palatoglossal seal (soft tongue-palate), very serious dysfunction that causes the fall of the bolus to the hypopharynx before the triggering of the decelerating motor pattern of the pharyngeal when the airway is still open, which leads to a predatory aspiration [15].

Videofluoroscopic Signs of the Pharyngeal Phase

The major videofluoroscopic signs of the efficacy of the pharyngeal phase are the hypopharyngeal residue and alterations opening of the upper esophageal sphincter (UES). A symmetric hypopharyngeal residue in both piriform sinuses is due to a weak pharyngeal contraction, very common in patients with neurodegenerative diseases, and predisposes post-swallowing aspiration. Patients with stroke may present a unilateral waste as a consequence of a unilateral pharyngeal paralysis. Video- fluoroscopic signs of safety of the pharyngeal phase are the slowness or the discoordination of the deglutory motor pattern pharyngeal and penetrations and/or aspirations (Fig. **1**). Penetration is the entry of contrast in the laryngeal vestibule without passing the vocal cords (Fig. **2**). If it produces an aspiration, the contrast goes through the vocal cords and it passes to the tracheobronchial tree (Fig. **3**). The possibility of digitization and quantitative analysis of images of video- fluoroscopy currently allows an accurate measurement of the oropharyngeal motor pattern in patients with dysphagia [16].

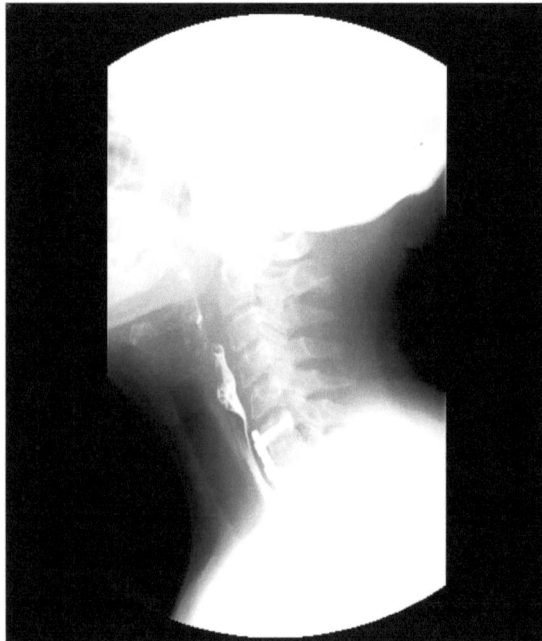

Fig. (1). Normal videofluoroscopic image.

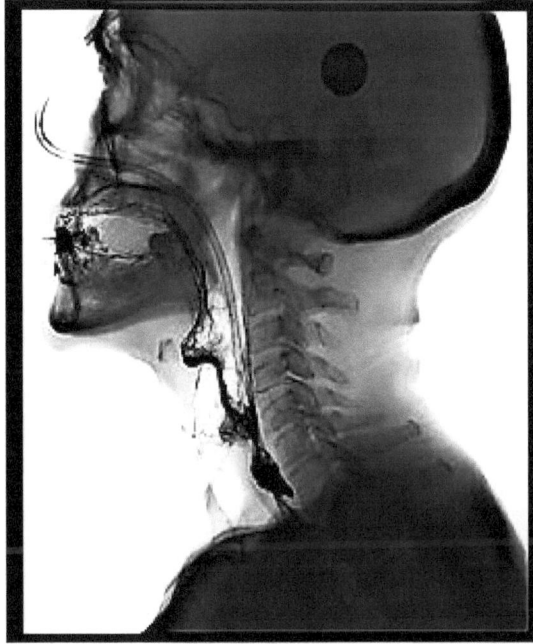

Fig. (2). Videofluoroscopic image with penetration in a patient with AD.

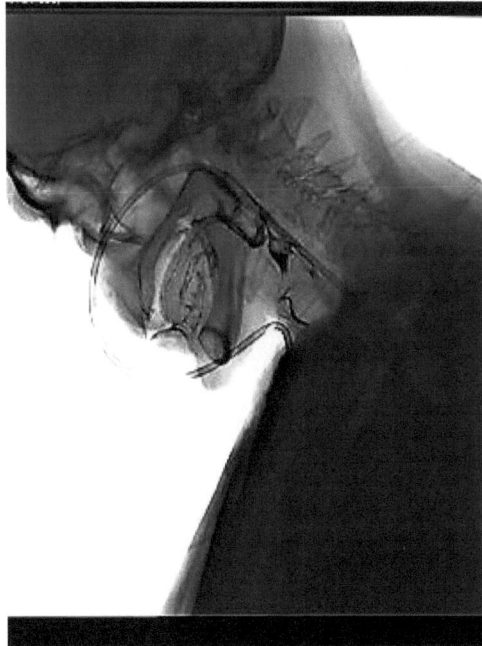

Fig. (3). Videofluoroscopic image of an AD patient with an aspiration.

Pharyngoesophageal Manometry

Pharyngoesophageal manometry is the technique of choice for the study of the mechanisms of opening of the UES. Some authors recommend performing the manometric and videofluoroscopic studies simultaneously (manofluorography).

Up to three patterns of alteration of the UES opening can be defined:

Decreased opening of the UES. It is caused by insufficient bolus propulsion, which is observed in up to 15% of patients with neurological or neuro-degenerative diseases and is characterized by a slow oropharyngeal motor response, a traction hyoid movement on the UES (early ascent and displacement) amplitude, weak bolus propulsion and strictly normal manometric relaxation. Many of these patients also present an alteration in the safety of swallowing in the form of penetrations or aspirations.

Incomplete neuromuscular relaxation of UES. It is observed in neurological diseases associated with spasticity of neural origin such as Parkinson's disease or traumatic brain injury. The pattern is characterized by a severe delay or even the absence of swallowing response, short hyoid movement, weak bolus propulsion and reduction or disappearance of neuromuscular relaxation and decrease in sphincter compliance in manometry.

Finally, the alteration of the ESS opening associated with Zenker's diverticulum [17].

TREATMENT OF DYSPHAGIA IN ALZHEIMER'S DISEASE

The goal of the treatment is maintenance of the oral route while it is possible to maintain nutritional status and avoid respiratory complications. The strategies of treatment of oropharyngeal dysphagia in Alzheimer's patients can be grouped into several categories: rehabilitative treatment (postural strategies, sensory increase, neuromuscular practices and specific maneuvers); modification of bolus characteristics; volume and viscosity; and percutaneous endoscopic gastrostomy. Additionally, dysphagia management requires a multidisciplinary approach considering that no single strategy is appropriate for all patients.

The current best clinical practice consists of the selection of the treatment according to the severity of the efficacy and safety alterations identified during the functional study: a) patients with discrete alterations of efficacy and a correct safety can follow a free diet; b) patients with moderate alterations require changes aimed at decreasing the volume and increasing the viscosity of the food bolus; c) patients with severe alterations also require strategies based on increased viscosity and the introduction of postural techniques, active maneuvers and oral sensory increase; and d) there is a group of patients with alterations so serious that it is not possible to treat them by the application of rehabilitation techniques, in which the oral route is not possible and it is necessary to evaluate the placement of a percutaneous endoscopic gastrostomy. Also we need dietary strategies to concentrate their caloric and protein requirements in the small volume of food they can eat [15].

Postural Strategies

They allow to modify the dimensions of the oropharynx and the path that the bolus should follow. The anterior flexion of the neck allows to protect the respiratory tract [18]; the posterior flexion facilitates pharyngeal gravitational drainage and improves oral transit speed; the rotation of the head towards the paralyzed pharyngeal side directs food to the healthy side, increases the effectiveness of pharyngeal transit and facilitates the opening of the UES; swallowing in lateral decubitus or in a supine position protects from aspiration of a hypopharyngeal residue. The effect of these strategies is modest, since they manage to avoid aspirations in 25% of patients where applied [19]. The atmosphere of the dining room, the interaction of the staff and the time dedicated to the feeding conditions affects the intake of residents. In general, care should be taken in oral hygiene, including taking care of teeth and prostheses, preserving the integrity of mucous membranes, lips and commissures. To minimize risks, the dining room environment should be relaxed, with the caretaker sitting at the same height as the patient, using verbal and body language appropriate to begin feeding patiently.

Oral Sensory Enhancement Strategies

It is preferable to use spoons rather than syringes, since they allow to observe the swallowing and the pressure in the tongue stimulates the swallowing reflex.

The spoon should approach from below and placed in the middle of the mouth pushing the tongue down to prevent it from retracting. Small amounts should be given at a time, preventing food from accumulating in the mouth and ensuring that the patient does not speak while eating.

We will leave enough time for swallowing, massaging the jaw or causing the patient to imitate our gestures if he does not open his mouth or chew. After each swallow, it is advisable to encourage him to cough and make sure the mouth is empty before administering the food again. If coughing occurs with swallowing, the feeding should be stopped. It is preferable to avoid straws and use low-mouth wide glasses. Particular attention must be paid to the presence of lumps, skins, *etc.*, which may remain in the purees. Remember also that acidic flavors and cold foods stimulate the mechanism of swallowing [20].

There are other less used techniques whose effectiveness still needs to be verified or require the patient to be cognitively intact and collaborative. These are rehabilitative exercises to improve swallowing (*e.g.* Shaker technique and Mendelsohn maneuver) and electrical stimulation.

Diet Modifications

The goal is to improve hydration and nutrition with safer swallowing and avoid complications such as bronchoaspiration. We must try to offer diets that are varied and attractive, while ensuring the adequate consumption of all food groups, which combine the needs of patient safety with the maintenance of the traditional taste for food.

As a general rule, we must avoid foods with different consistencies (pasta soups, milk with cereals), sticky foods (honey, chocolate), fibrous (pineapple, asparagus), fruits or vegetables with skin or pips (grapes, strawberries, kiwis, tomato), foods that produce sialorrhea (candy) or that release water or juice when biting or crushing.

The rations should be smaller and, taking into account that the swallowing time is increased by 2-4 times, it is necessary to program more doses that do not exceed 45 minutes distributed throughout the 24 hours.

The main alternatives for the modification of the texture of the food are:

-Crushed solid foods (crushed diet) / lyophilized products

-Use of texture modifiers: thickeners and jellies...

-Enrichment of the diet: food, modules and supplementation.

In patients with Alzheimer's disease and dysphagia, the reduction of bolus volume and viscosity increases improves efficacy and safety, with a significant drop in penetrations and aspirations.

These changes in volume and viscosity of the bolus are a very valuable therapeutic strategy, since it is a method that does not fatigue, does not require cognitive integrity and does not involve any learning, and the application of the strategy is in the charge of the caregiver [6, 15].

Oral Supplementation

Due to the characteristics of patients with Alzheimer's disease, it is common for the patient to not reach the desirable energy requirements.

To achieve this energy supply, it is possible to add nutritional oral supplements to the crushed diet. But we have to bear in mind that they are usually marketed with liquid texture, therefore, thickeners should be used to improve safety in swallowing.

Percutaneous Endoscopic Gastrostomy

When an individual with Alzheimer's disease reaches de advanced stages of the disease and is no longer able to eat, even with assistance, when the risk of nutritional decline and aspiration pneumonia is high, we normally propose to insert a feeding tube for artificial nutrition and hydration. This irreversible stage is the expected course of AD.

It is very controversial whether tube feeding in people with dementia (Alzheimer's disease included) improves nutritional status or prolongs survival. Guidelines published by several professional societies cite observational studies that have shown no benefit and conclude that tube feeding in patients with advanced dementia should be avoided.

In general, the results of studies in terms of tube feeding do not show an improvement in nutritional status, nor that they prevent or reduce the incidence of aspiration pneumonia, nor that pressure ulcers decrease. There is also no data to support greater survival among patients with advanced Alzheimer's who are tube-fed compared to careful manual feeding. As drawbacks of tube feeding we have the increased need to use physical restraint measures to prevent patients from withdrawing tubes. Another drawback is the deprivation of savoring the food and the contact that is received from the caregiver at the moments of the help in the feeding.

However, some authors suggest that all the studies on tube feeding in dementia have important methodological flaws that invalidate their findings. The current evidence is not sufficient to justify general guidelines. Patients with advanced dementia represent a very heterogeneous group, and evidence shows that some patients with dementia benefit from tube feeding [21].

We should not prematurely take tube feeding off the table as an option. A comprehensive presentation of its benefits and potential burdens should be presented to patients (or their surrogates) for their own determination [22].

We think that the aim must be an improvement in the quality of life, not a prolongation of terminal disease [23].

We need to keep in mind that there are absolute contraindications of percutaneous endoscopic gastrostomy (PEG): the inability to perform a gastroscopy (esophageal strictures), ascites, gastric cancer, coagulopathies, gastric bleeding, partial or total gastrectomy, infection of the abdominal wall and severe disorders of intestinal motility.

The relative contraindications are a large hiatal hernia, non-resective gastric surgery, and the impossibility of transillumination due to obesity, kyphoscoliosis or transposition of the colon.

The most common mild complications of PEG are local stoma infection, which is usually resolved with local treatment, and bleeding, which is usually self-limiting. Occasionally (1-4%) there may be serious complications such as abdominal infections, bleeding, perforation and pneumoperitoneum, secondary to accidental and early catheter extraction [24, 25].

In conclusion, decisions regarding tube feeding can be extremely difficult for caregivers and/or surrogates. It is very important that health staff assist the caregivers in the decision-making process and offer alternatives to tube feeding that demonstrate care and compassion to the person with AD. We have to emphasize that careful hand feeding offers the highest quality of care and should be offered to all individuals with advanced AD who can competently and comfortably handle oral feeding. Before reaching this stage, individuals with AD should discuss this and other end-of-life decisions with their care partners, including their physician, early in the course of the disease. Then, when they reach this advanced stages, the caregivers and surrogates can respect the wishes of the patient, a situation that does not always happen [26].

CONSENT FOR PUBLICATION

Not applicable.

ACKNOWLEDGEMENTS

Declared none

CONFLICT OF INTEREST

The authors confirm that this chapter contents have no conflict of interest.

REFERENCES

[1]   Easterling CS, Robbins E. Dementia and dysphagia. Geriatr Nurs 2008; 29(4): 275-85.
       [http://dx.doi.org/10.1016/j.gerinurse.2007.10.015] [PMID: 18694703]

[2]   Chouinard J. Dysphagia in Alzheimer disease: a review. J Nutr Health Aging 2000; 4(4): 214-7.
       [PMID: 11115803]

[3]   Martin RE, Sessle BJ. The role of the cerebral cortex in swallowing. Dysphagia 1993; 8(3): 195-202.
       [http://dx.doi.org/10.1007/BF01354538] [PMID: 8359039]

[4]   Gómez-Busto F, Atares B, Moreno V. Correlación clínico-patológica de los diagnósticos de muerte en una residencia mixta. Rev Esp Geriatr Gerontol 2001; 36: 3.

[5]   Humbert IA, McLaren DG, Kosmatka K, *et al.* Early deficits in cortical control of swallowing in Alzheimer's disease. J Alzheimers Dis 2010; 19(4): 1185-97.
       [http://dx.doi.org/10.3233/JAD-2010-1316] [PMID: 20308785]

[6]   Gómez-Busto F, Andia V, Ruiz de Alegría L, Francés I. Abordaje de la disfagia en la demencia avanzada. Rev Esp Geriatr Gerontol 2009; 44 (Suppl. 2): 29-36.
       [http://dx.doi.org/10.1016/j.regg.2008.07.006] [PMID: 19800150]

[7]   Sato E1, Hirano H, Watanabe Y. Detecting signs of dysphagia in patients with Alzheimer's disease with oral feeding in daily life. Geriatr Gerontol Int 2014 Jul; 14 (3): 549-55.

[8]   Satoshi HORIGUCHI, Yasushi SUZUKI. Screening tests in evaluating swallowing function. JMAJ 2011; 54(1): 31-4.

[9]   Kubota T, Mishima H, Hanada M, *et al.* Paralytic dysphagia in cerebrovascular disorder—screening tests and their clinical application. General Rehabilitation 1982; 10: 271-6.

[10]   Takahashi K. Cervical auscultation. Eating and Swallowing Rehabilitation. Tokyo: Ishiyaku Publishers 1998; pp. 171-5.

[11]   Clavé P, Almirall J, Esteve M, *et al.* Dysphagia – a team approach to prevent and treat complications. Hospital Healthcare Europe 2005/2006. Campden Publishing Ltd (eds). 2005; pp. N5-8.

[12]   Sherman B, Nisenboum JM, Jesberger BL, Morrow CA, Jesberger JA. Assessment of dysphagia with the use of pulse oximetry. Dysphagia 1999; 14(3): 152-6.
       [http://dx.doi.org/10.1007/PL00009597] [PMID: 10341112]

[13]   Clavé P. Métodos de estudio de la neurofisiología de la deglución y de la disfagia orofaríngea. Rev Esp Enferm Dig 2004; 96 (Suppl. 2): 47-9.

[14]   Clavé P. Videofluoroscopic diagnosis of oropharyngeal dysphagia. Nutrition Matters 2001; 3: 1-2.

[15]   Clavé P, Arreola V, Velasco M, *et al.* Diagnóstico y tratamiento de la disfagia orofaríngea funcional. Aspectos de interés para el cirujano digestivo. Cir Esp 2007; 82(2): 62-76.
       [http://dx.doi.org/10.1016/S0009-739X(07)71672-X] [PMID: 17785140]

[16]   Clavé P, de Kraa M, Arreola V, *et al.* The effect of bolus viscosity on swallowing function in neurogenic dysphagia. Aliment Pharmacol Ther 2006; 24(9): 1385-94.
       [http://dx.doi.org/10.1111/j.1365-2036.2006.03118.x] [PMID: 17059520]

[17]   Clavé P, Terré R, de Kraa M, Serra M. Approaching oropharyngeal dysphagia. Rev Esp Enferm Dig 2004; 96(2): 119-31.
       [http://dx.doi.org/10.4321/S1130-01082004000200005] [PMID: 15255021]

[18]   Rasley A, Logemann JA, Kahrilas PJ, Rademaker AW, Pauloski BR, Dodds WJ. Prevention of barium aspiration during videofluoroscopic swallowing studies: value of change in posture. AJR Am J Roentgenol 1993; 160(5): 1005-9.
       [http://dx.doi.org/10.2214/ajr.160.5.8470567] [PMID: 8470567]

[19]   Logemann JA, Kahrilas PJ, Kobara M, Vakil NB. The benefit of head rotation on pharyngoesophageal dysphagia. Arch Phys Med Rehabil 1989; 70(10): 767-71.

[PMID: 2802957]

[20] Bisch EM, Logemann JA, Rademaker AW, Kahrilas PJ, Lazarus CL. Pharyngeal effects of bolus volume, viscosity, and temperature in patients with dysphagia resulting from neurologic impairment and in normal subjects. J Speech Hear Res 1994; 37(5): 1041-59.
[http://dx.doi.org/10.1044/jshr.3705.1041] [PMID: 7823550]

[21] Feeding issues in Advanced Dementia. From alz.org. Alzheimer's association. 2015. Available from: https://www.alz.org/documents_custom/statements/Feeding_Issues.pdf

[22] Lynch MC. Is tube feeding futile in advanced dementia? Linacre Q 2016; 83(3): 283-307.
[http://dx.doi.org/10.1080/00243639.2016.1211879] [PMID: 27833208]

[23] Pennington C. To PEG or not to PEG. Clin Med (Lond) 2002; 2(3): 250-5.
[http://dx.doi.org/10.7861/clinmedicine.2-3-250] [PMID: 12108477]

[24] Mellinger JD, Ponsky JL. Percutaneous endoscopic gastrostomy. Endoscopy 1994; 26(1): 55-9.
[http://dx.doi.org/10.1055/s-2007-1005810] [PMID: 8205997]

[25] Schapiro GD, Edmundowicz SA. Complications of percutaneous endoscopic gastrostomy. Gastrointest Endosc Clin N Am 1996; 6(2): 409-22.
[http://dx.doi.org/10.1016/S1052-5157(18)30369-6] [PMID: 8673334]

[26] White GN, O'Rourke F, Ong BS, Cordato DJ, Chan DK. Dysphagia: causes, assessment, treatment, and management. Geriatrics 2008; 63(5): 15-20.
[PMID: 18447407]

CHAPTER 5

Biomarkers for the Diagnosis of Alzheimer's Disease

Francisco J. Barrero Hernández[*]

Service of Neurology, "San Cecilio" Hospital. University of Granada, Granada, Spain

Abstract: Neurodegeneration in Alzheimer's disease starts several years before clinical manifestations are present; they make it possible to establish the clinical diagnosis of the disease. In this continuum of neurodegeneration there are still unknown factors to solve, although much progress has been made in identifying neuropathological, biochemical and genetic signs that help to diagnose the disease in the early stages (mild cognitive impairment) in order to start earlier an effective treatment.

There are several biomarkers proposed for the diagnosis of Alzheimer's disease such as neuroimaging with measurement of brain atrophy; also those related to glucose tracers, beta-amyloid and tau protein in (PET) Positron Emission Tomography; and in recent years, cerebrospinal fluid with the determination of beta-amyloid, tau, p-Tau and other proteins is being studied.

Keywords: Alzheimer´s Disease, β Amyloid, Biomarkers, Dementia, Cerebrospinal Fluid, Neuroimaging, PET, RMI, Tau.

INTRODUCTION

Alzheimer disease (AD) is a neurodegenerative disease in which molecular lesions produce loss of neurons, synapse, and gliosis with a subsequent cognitive and behavioral impairment resulting in alteration of patient autonomy. The main risk factor for the AD is aging; more than 90% occur in individuals older than 65. The increasing age of the population will probably lead to the increase of the incidence of the disease in the coming years, with an important social and economic impact. Other risk factors associated with AD are a family history of the disease, cerebrovascular disease and other cardiovascular risk factors (hypertension, diabetes mellitus), chronic inflammation, brain trauma, sleep apnea and poor schooling [1 - 5]. The most frequent type of dementia is AD; more than

[*] **Corresponding author Francisco J. Barrero Hernández:** Service of Neurology, "Campus de la Salud" Hospital, University of Granada, Spain; Tel: 677224436; E-mail: fjbarreroh@ugr.es

Blas Gil-Extremera (Ed.)
All rights reserved-© 2019 Bentham Science Publishers

45 million people are diagnosed with probable AD, and 130 million people could have mild cognitive impairment due to the disease [6].

According to the latest update of the diagnosis of AD by the National Institute on Aging-Alzheimer's Association of 2011 [7], AD is diagnosed when there are cognitive and behavioral changes (with two domains affected, one of them being the memory) of insidious onset and progressive course and a decrease in functionality from the previous state. Excluding other non degenerative causes, primary psychiatric disorders, or systemic alterations. At the beginning of the first symptoms it is difficult and not always possible to establish a diagnosis only based on clinical features and the evolution of the symptoms. Definitive diagnosis is carried out through histopathological studies. According to the clinical practice, neuroimaging, genetic and molecular biomarkers are essential in the early and accurate diagnosis of the disease, excluding the most common and treatable secondary causes of AD such as hypothyroidism, vitamin B12 deficiency, infections or drug and toxic causes. The application of biomarkers is already included in the new criteria: magnetic resonance imaging (MRI), 18F-fluorodeoxyglucose positron emission tomography (18-FDG-PET), PET amyloid imaging study and amyloid marker in the cerebrospinal fluid (CSF) [7]. The diagnosis of AD becomes clear, when clinical symptoms are present in all their magnitude. But as in any degenerative disease, the onset of the disease presents with minimal, subjective and even non-specific clinical symptoms. There are different clinical phenotypes within the spectrum of the EA: amnesic mild cognitive impairment, focal variants (logopenic variant, posterior atrophy), and even asymptomatic patients with a family history of early onset of the disease. In these cases, biomarkers are essential in the early and more accurate diagnosis of AD.

PATHOGENESIS

AD is postulated as a dual proteinopathy according to the hypothesis of amyloidogenic and hyperphosphorylated tau protein hypothesis.

Subjects with AD present beta amyloid protein aggregates in the brain tissue. β-amyloid is a peptide of 35-43 amino acids resulting from the spin-off of the amyloid precursor protein (APP) by the beta and gamma secretases forming flexible and soluble oligomers that can be metabolized. Sometimes oligomers produce errors inducing beta-amyloid plaques, which cannot be cleared, accumulating in the brain. β amyloid 42 (Aβ42) is the most frequent isoform in the neuritic or senile plaque [8].

P-tau protein (abnormal) does not bind to microtubules due to a misfolding, then forming insoluble fibrillar neurofilaments. Tau is involved in neuronal signaling pathways and eventually premature apoptosis occurs. The hyperphosphorylation of microtubule-associated tau protein leads to neuronal death [9].

In AD, extracellular protein aggregates of Ab42 fibrins and to a lesser extent Ab40 fibrins coexist, which form β-amyloid neuritic plaques, and intracellular aggregates of hyperphosphorylated tau (p-Tau), producing neurofibrillary tangles [10, 11].

The spread of neurofibrillary tangles in AD was described by Braak in four stages [12]. This distribution of p-Tau correlates better than a diffuse amyloid deposition, with the progression of cognitive symptoms, at the time of the presentation of symptoms [12]. Clinical and anatomic correlations are produced by the p-Tau protein deposition, with subcortical onset in the noradrenergic neurons of the locus coeruleus, which exends to the limbic system. Other regions with p-Tau deposition are cholinergic neurons of the nucleus basalis of Meynert and serotonergic neurons in the dorsal Raphe nucleus. The first regions with tau protein aggregates include the trans enthorinal cortex, medial temporal lobe, hippocampus and the anterior and basal part of the brain (forebrain) followed by the allocortex and the rest of the neocortex [13].

BIOMARKERS IN ALZHEIMER'S DISEASE

A biomarker is a characteristic that can be objectively measured and evaluated as an indicator of normal biological process, pathological process or pharmacological response to therapeutic intervention [14].

The applications of biomarkers in such neurodegenerative diseases as AD can help us in the daily clinical practice: (1) in the diagnosis at early stages of disease in subjects participating in clinical trials; (2) as diagnostic tool associated with the differential diagnosis; (3) in the clinical staging of the disease; (4) as indicator in the disease prognosis; and (5) in monitoring the response to treatments [15].

Let's not forget the utility of biomarkers in research to a better understanding of the mechanisms involved in the pathogenesis and pathophysiology of AD, not only in animal models, but also in our patients.

There are several biomarkers proposed for the diagnosis of AD. Neuroimaging with measurement of brain atrophy; also those related to glucose tracers, β-amyloid and tau protein in positron emission tomography (PET) [2].

In recent years, the study of CSF with the determination of beta-amyloid, tau, p-Tau and other proteins is essential, with very relevant findings concerning the pathogenesis of the disease [3].

Except for PET studies, which have been validated with necropsy studies of patients [16 - 18], the study of biomarkers in CSF has only been validated with PET [19].

We summarize the different biomarkers (Table **1**) with greater clinical application in AD, classified as: genetic, biochemical, and neuroimaging biomarkers.

Table 1. Biomarkers in AD.

Biomarkers in AD	
GENETIC	
APOE-ε4	Homozygote
PPA	Chromosome 21
PSEN1	Chromosome 14
PSEN2	Chromosome 1
CSF	
β42 amyloid	↓ Concentration
Aβ42/Aβ40 ratio	↓ Ratio
p-tau, t-tau	↑ Concentration
NEUROIMAGING	
MR 3D T1 weighted	↓ Volume of hippocampus and medial temporal structures
PET 18-FDG	↓ Metabolism in posterior cingulate-precuneus and temporoparietal cortex
PET 11C-Pittsburgh Compound B	↑ cortex deposition
PET amiloide	↑ uptake is typically diffuse in the neocortex
PET tau	↑ uptake

AD: Alzheimer´s disease; CFS: cerebrospinal fluid; APP: amyloid precursor protein; PSEN1: presenilin-1; PSEN2: presenilin-2; p-tau: fosfo-tau; t-tau: tau total; FDG: fluorodeoxyglucose, PET 11C-Pitsburgh Compound B: 18F ligands (Cortical uptake Brain Amyloidosis AD)

Genetic Biomarkers

There are families with a high incidence of AD in their members. An early clinical onset is characteristic. Autosomal dominant forms represent less than 2% of all patients with AD. It is estimated that of these types genetically complex of AD with an early onset, only 10-20% of the subjects with a family history of AD present a Mendelian inheritance pattern. The genes usually involved in these forms are the gene of amyloid precursor protein (APP) on chromosome 21, presenilin-1 (PSEN1) on chromosome 14, and presenilin-2 (PSEN2) on chromosome 1 with dominant autosomal inheritance. These mutated genes contribute to the increase of Aβ42, to the amyloid formation and inflammation [20].

In the sporadic forms, the ε4 allele of apolipoprotein E (APOE-ε4) in homozygous state continues to be the most frequently associated to AD, with and increase of risk of 15 times compared with the heterozygous presentation [21]. About 20 genetic variants of risk and protection with a very discreet individual influence by GWAS studies have been identified [22].

Biochemical Biomarkers

These markers can be obtained from different fluids. We analyzed the markers obtained in CSF and plasma, although the latter are still pending to demonstrate their clinical validity; there are still no data reliably demonstrated.

Biomarkers in CSF

Amyloid β protein in CSF: Amyloid β protein can be determined in CSF by dependent antibodies such as enzyme-linked immunosorbent assay (ELISA) or mass spectrometry. Concentrations of amyloid β42 protein are found to be decreased not only in patients with AD, but also in mild cognitive impairment and preclinical phase of the disease [23]. This decrease is consistent with the aggregation, in the (senile) neuritic plaques in patients, as probed in autopsy studies and *in vivo* amyloid PET study [24].

To ensure that the data obtained from CSF are valid, it must be taken into account that the patients have not had any episode of stroke, head trauma or meningitis at least 3-6 months before fluid biomarker is performed in order not to alter the results [25].

Tau- protein in CSF: Neurofibrillary tangles in AD are mainly formed by p-Tau protein; their function is to stabilize the microtubules in axons. The concentration of p-Tau is elevated in subjects with AD. A correlation has been found between the concentration of p-Tau and the study of tau-PET neuroimaging studies [26].

An increase of p-Tau in CSF has not been demonstrated consistently in other tauopathies, such as progressive supranuclear palsy (PSP) or frontotemporal dementias (FTD). However, several data have been published of p-Tau in other diseases, such as herpes virus encephalitis [27], and superficial siderosis [28].

Total tau (t-tau) protein, formed by non phosphorylated sequences is elevated in the CSF of patients with AD [23] and correlates positively with neurodegenerative intensity [29]. The specificity of t-tau is not complete as it has been found in Creutzfeldt-Jakob disease (CJD) or after a stroke episode [25]. Many studies have demonstrated that even in early stages of AD, there is an increase in the concentrations of tau-protein and a decrease in the concentrations of beta amyloid (1-42) b1-42 in CSF [30, 31]. The diagnostic accuracy of AD in these biomarkers reaches 80% - 95% [32].

At present, the most reliable biomarkers proposed are those obtained in CSF, by measuring the levels of Aβ42, total tau and phospho-tau. A decrease in the concentration of Aβ42 is found in the early stages of the disease, as well as an increase in tau and p-Tau [33]. The relationship between Aβ42/Aβ40 shows a better correlation with the amyloid deposition in mild cognitive impairment, and it is a more reliable marker of AD compared to other dementias [34]. Given the diversity of studies in relation to biomarkers in CSF in AD, some experts agree with the recommendations when interpreting the results of biomarkers in CSF of our patients and always taking into account the clinical features, since sometimes the results can be ambiguous [35].

Biomarkers in Plasma

Given the discomfort and the risk, although minimum, of complications when making lumbar puncture for the study of CSF, tau protein and Aβ42 in plasma have been studied.

Plasma concentrations of β amyloid do not correlate with the data obtained in CSF, in part because of its influence in the production at the peripheral level by platelets and other extracerebral tissues [36].

There is an interaction of Aβ42 determinations in plasma with drugs such as insulin [37]. Plasma T-tau levels are increased, but less than in the CSF of patients with AD, and it has not been demonstrated to be increased in mild cognitive impairment [38].

The data obtained are not conclusive, due in part to the low concentrations of these markers (tau and Aβ42) in plasma. Several techniques have been proposed to detect ultra-high sensitivity proteins using superconducting-quantu--interference - device (SQUID) using immunomagnetic reduction (SQUID-based IMR) assay, that allow to measure plasma proteins although concentrations are minimal as in the case of AD biomarkers in plasma.

IMR applied to patients with MCI due to AD and early stages of AD provides accuracy of 85% in diagnosis in relation to the concentration levels of tau and Aβ142. Authors reported the low cost and low risk to the patient of the blood test [39].

Biomarkers in Saliva

Some authors have studied the determination of beta-amyloid 1-42 and Tau in saliva of patients with AD [40, 41]. Lactoferrin in saliva has been proposed as a biomarker for MCI and AD. This peptide secreted in saliva has an important antimicrobial effect against bacteria, fungi, viruses, and yeasts [42]. Its activity has been associated to the modulatory effect of the immune response; it is well known the theory of the association of amyloid aggregation with infections [43]. Carro and colleagues determined low levels of lactoferrin in a cohort of patients clinically diagnosed with an amnestic cognitive impairment and AD compared with healthy controls [44].They also obtained correlation with the CSF biomarkers (Aβ42 and t-tau protein). Further studies about the validation data in subjects with DFT and mild cognitive dementia are needed. However, today a validation study with neuroimaging PET and CSF markers is being carried out. The preliminary results show some promise.

Other Biomarkers in CSF for AD

The ratio between albumin in CSF and serum gives an idea of the integrity of the blood-brain barrier, which is not increased in AD, in contrast what happens in patients with vascular dementia [45].

Visinin-like protein 1 (VLP-1), fatty acid-binding protein (FABP), and neuron-specific enolase (NSE) are molecules associated in part to AD, but in a weak form compared to t-tau [23].

The light neurofilaments (NF-L) have been found to be elevated in AD, especially in forms more rapidly progressive [46]. A high concentration is also found in DFT, CJD, vascular dementia and atypical parkinsonism [25]. However, some authors showed an increase of tau protein and neurofilaments in plasma in patients with AD; these results being comparable with the CSF biomarkers in the prediction of future cognitive impairment [47]. Neurogranin (Ng), as dendritic protein related to the synapse, is found to be elevated in the CSF of patients with AD. There are already references that related it to the prediction of cognitive impairment, and cerebral atrophy in EA [48].

Structural Biomarkers (Neuroimaging)

It is well known the classic studies of morphological neuroimaging using computed tomography and magnetic resonance imaging (MRI), both useful in measuring the degree of cerebral atrophy in specific regions of the hippocampus, entorhinal cortex, corpus callosum and other areas early involved in AD [49].

Other neuroimaging techniques such as fluorodeoxyglucose positron emission tomography (FDG PET), affecting the medial temporal lobe, medial parietal lobe (precuneus), posterior cingulate cortex, and temporo-parietal association cortex must be also considered [50]. Some studies show a sensitivity of 94% and 73% specificity for predicting the clinical outcome and diagnosis of AD. So a negative PET predicted that in the following 3 years, it was unlikely that a clinical evolution to AD occurs [51].

At present, there are specific radioligand that are directly associated with β-amyloid plaques and tau protein, or both, that allow the display of these abnormal proteins *in vivo.*

One of these is the *Pittsburgh Compound-B* (PiB), an analog of thioflavin, selective for β-amyloid plaques. This compound is used only in research. In neuroimaging studies, subjects with AD present a retention of PiB between 60-90% higher than controls. This deposit is correlated with the levels of β-amyloid [52].

In the clinical practice, we already have the possibility to carry out amyloid PET using tracers such as the florbetapir, flutemetamol and florbetaben [53]. Postmortem studies are done to demonstrate tau protein deposition, which has been correlated with cognitive dysfunction [54] and cortical patterns similar to those described by Braak [10] with flortaucipir [55, 56].

Other authors have also demonstrated the concordance between the results of FDG-PET, (Aβ42), and p-Tau in CSF [57]. PET presents some limitations, as evidenced in subjects in the preclinical phase in which the density of neuritic plaques is low, which can lead to obtain a false negative with amyloid-PET; it is not a suitable method in the selection of patients for anti-amyloid therapies.

In a series of 2332 autopsies of the brain, Braak and colleagues, found neurofibrillary tangles (p-Tau) in the absence of amyloid in the first stages of AD [58]. In the course of the disease, there is a plateau in the density of beta amyloid, which can limit the interpretation when the density of neuritic plaques is reduced [59]. So far, in phase III clinical trials with solanezumab and bapineuzumab, the reduction of beta amyloid load reduction is not accompanied by the improvement of clinical cognitive function [60]. Although there are promising data about a correlation with clinical improvement using aducanumab [61].

THE NEED FOR BIOMARKERS IN ALZHEIMER'S DISEASE

The possibility of obtaining *in vivo* biomarkers in subjects with AD, leads not only to improve the diagnostic success in the clinical suspicion of the disease.

According to the natural history of the disease and taking into account degeneration in AD models, a preclinical stage exists [62]. AD biomarkers will help to know and determine those subjects with an early onset of the disease. However, we have to think about the limitations of the diagnosis in the preclinical phase, without having today an effective treatment that might change the course of the disease. Neurodegeneration is a continuous process (Fig. **1**) [70] going from the preclinical stage, asymptomatic stage (mild cognitive impairment) and finally, dementia [63].

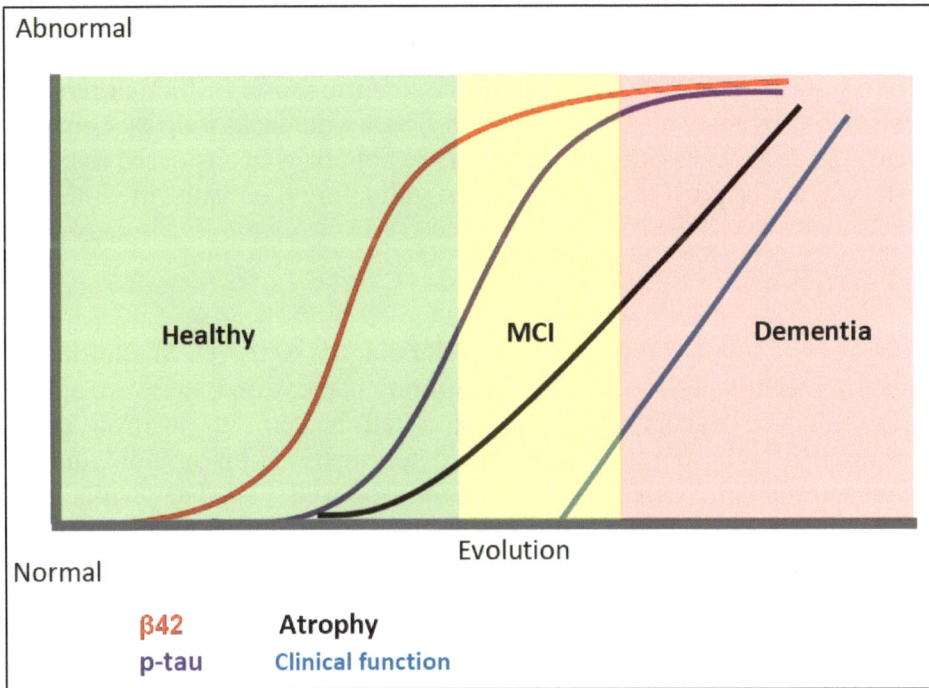

Fig. (1). Evolution of Biomarkers in Alzheimer's Disease.

Biomarkers can be used in the early stages of the pathogenetic process to change the course of the disease using the current drugs available, and certainly with more success with future treatments, avoiding the accumulation of abnormal protein aggregates in neurons and glia that lead to irreversible damage. The possibility that biomarkers, mainly those with molecular specificity for AD, becomes a reality in the clinical practice, can help bridging the so-called "Valley of Death" [64] where the rate of drugs approved for the treatment of AD is null. So far, anticholinesterase is available some years ago (Donepezil, rivastigmine and galantamine) and memantine as blocker of excitotoxicity glutamatergic was approved by the FDA in 2003.

CLINICAL UTILITY OF BIOMARKERS

In the daily clinical practice, biomarkers help to determine the clinical diagnosis or the stage of the disease. Obviously the interpretation of the results depends on the clinical phenotype. The utility of biomarkers decreases with age, since the incidence of asymptomatic AD increases dramatically in people aged 70 or older. A better diagnostic performance, has been proposed a combined application of clinical assessment, CSF, and neuroimaging markers, such as with an AUC of 0.96 for patients with a conversion from MCI to AD [65]. The risk of this conversion has also been demonstrated with 18F-FDG-PET and 11 c-GDP-PET either individually or using both markers with an AUC of 0.89 and 0.81, respectively [66]. Although advances in the determination of biomarkers for the diagnosis and prognosis of AD are booming, today the lack of disease-modifying treatments for AD makes these biomarkers are not always considered as essential, although they are of great importance when validating the results in clinical trials [67].

CONCLUSIONS

There are several biomarkers proposed in the diagnosis of AD. In addition to the neuroimaging techniques by which brain atrophy is measured, there are also those related to glucose tracers, β-amyloid and tau protein in positron emission tomography (PET) [2]. In recent years, the determination of β-amyloid, tau, p-Tau and other proteins in CSF has also been proposed [3]. The availability of biomarkers that showed a correlation with clinical data of cognitive impairment and specific neuroimaging markers represents a major breakthrough to increase the diagnostic certainty, mainly in the early stages of the disease.

Today in clinical practice, biomarkers are used in subjects with an early onset of AD, or in the presence of atypical signs, such as rapid progression, severe behavioral impairment or associated motor disorders. In subjects with late onset of the disease, structural neuroimaging provides information on the involvement of other associated factors: cerebrovascular disease or the possibility of alternative diagnosis, such as stroke or neoplasia.

The concentration of tau protein appears in the early course of the disease; its close association with the severity of neurodegeneration has led to consider AD as a tauopathy.

P-tau in CSF is currently considered the most specific biomarker in the diagnosis of AD. The possibility of combining Aβ42 t-tau improves the sensitivity and specificity, mainly the ratio Aβ42 and p-Tau (88% and 90%, respectively) in the prediction of conversion to AD [68]. Despite all the published scientific evidence, further studies are needed to expand the knowledge and the validation of biomarkers in order to propose those especially useful in the daily clinical practice. It is necessary to establish the roadmap taking into account the local and specific circumstances in each health system. The availability of these techniques in the clinical practice must avoid the over diagnosis of subjects without AD and, therefore, avoid the inappropriate treatment of these patients [69].

CONSENT FOR PUBLICATION

Not applicable.

ACKNOWLEDGEMENTS

Declare none.

CONFLICT OF INTEREST

The author confirms that this chapter content has no conflict of interest.

REFERENCES

[1]   Jansen WJ, Ossenkoppele R, Knol DL, *et al.* Prevalence of cerebral amyloid pathology in persons without dementia: a meta-analysis. JAMA 2015; 313(19): 1924-38.
        [http://dx.doi.org/10.1001/jama.2015.4668] [PMID: 25988462]

[2]   Villemagne VL, Doré V, Bourgeat P, *et al.* Abeta-amyloid and Tau imaging in dementia. Semin Nucl Med 2017; 47(1): 75-88.
        [http://dx.doi.org/10.1053/j.semnuclmed.2016.09.006] [PMID: 27987560]

[3]   Höglund K, Kern S, Zettergren A, *et al.* Preclinical amyloid pathology biomarker positivity: effects on tau pathology and neurodegeneration. Transl Psychiatry 2017; 7(1): e995.
        [http://dx.doi.org/10.1038/tp.2016.252] [PMID: 28072416]

[4]   Baumgart M, Snyder HM, Carrillo MC, Fazio S, Kim H, Johns H. Summary of the evidence on modifiable risk factors for cognitive decline and dementia: A population-based perspective. Alzheimers Dement 2015; 11(6): 718-26.
        [http://dx.doi.org/10.1016/j.jalz.2015.05.016] [PMID: 26045020]

[5]   Osorio RS, Gumb T, Pirraglia E, *et al.* Sleep-disordered breathing advances cognitive decline in the elderly. Neurology 2015; 84(19): 1964-71.
        [http://dx.doi.org/10.1212/WNL.0000000000001566] [PMID: 25878183]

[6]   Alzheimer's Association. Alzheimer's disease facts and figures. Alzheimers Dement 2015; 11: 332-84.https://www.alz.co.uk/research/statistics
        [PMID: 25984581]

[7]   McKhann GM, Knopman DS, Chertkow H, *et al.* The diagnosis of dementia due to Alzheimer's disease: recommendations from the National Institute on Aging-Alzheimer's Association workgroups on diagnostic guidelines for Alzheimer's disease. Alzheimers Dement 2011; 7(3): 263-9.
        [http://dx.doi.org/10.1016/j.jalz.2011.03.005] [PMID: 21514250]

[8]   Hardy JA, Higgins GA. Alzheimer's disease: the amyloid cascade hypothesis. Science 1992; 256(5054): 184-5.
        [http://dx.doi.org/10.1126/science.1566067] [PMID: 1566067]

[9]   de Calignon A, Polydoro M, Suárez-Calvet M, *et al.* Propagation of tau pathology in a model of early Alzheimer's disease. Neuron 2012; 73(4): 685-97.
[http://dx.doi.org/10.1016/j.neuron.2011.11.033] [PMID: 22365544]

[10]   Braak H, Braak E. Neuropathological stageing of Alzheimer-related changes. Acta Neuropathol 1991; 82(4): 239-59.
[http://dx.doi.org/10.1007/BF00308809] [PMID: 1759558]

[11]   Taylor JP, Hardy J, Fischbeck KH. Toxic proteins in neurodegenerative disease. Science 2002; 296(5575): 1991-5.
[http://dx.doi.org/10.1126/science.1067122] [PMID: 12065827]

[12]   Braak H, Alafuzoff I, Arzberger T, Kretzschmar H, Del Tredici K. Staging of Alzheimer disease-associated neurofibrillary pathology using paraffin sections and immunocytochemistry. Acta Neuropathol 2006; 112(4): 389-404.
[http://dx.doi.org/10.1007/s00401-006-0127-z] [PMID: 16906426]

[13]   Grudzien A, Shaw P, Weintraub S, Bigio E, Mash DC, Mesulam MM. Locus coeruleus neurofibrillary degeneration in aging, mild cognitive impairment and early Alzheimer's disease. Neurobiol Aging 2007; 28(3): 327-35.
[http://dx.doi.org/10.1016/j.neurobiolaging.2006.02.007] [PMID: 16574280]

[14]   Jain KK. Biomarkers of neurological disorders.Applications of Biotechnology in Neurology. Totowa, NJ: Humana Press 2012; pp. 49-53.

[15]   Beach TG, Beach A. A review of biomarkers for neurodegenerative disease: Will They Swing Us Across the Valley? Neurol Ther 2017; 6 (Suppl. 1): 5-13.
[http://dx.doi.org/10.1007/s40120-017-0072-x] [PMID: 28733961]

[16]   Sabri O, Sabbagh MN, Seibyl J, *et al.* Florbetaben PET imaging to detect amyloid beta plaques in Alzheimer's disease: phase 3 study. Alzheimers Dement 2015; 11(8): 964-74.
[http://dx.doi.org/10.1016/j.jalz.2015.02.004] [PMID: 25824567]

[17]   Clark CM, Pontecorvo MJ, Beach TG, *et al.* Cerebral PET with florbetapir compared with neuropathology at autopsy for detection of neuritic amyloid-β plaques: a prospective cohort study. Lancet Neurol 2012; 11(8): 669-78.
[http://dx.doi.org/10.1016/S1474-4422(12)70142-4] [PMID: 22749065]

[18]   Curtis C, Gámez JE, Singh U, *et al.* Phase 3 trial of flutemetamol labeled with radioactive fluorine 18 imaging and neuritic plaque density. JAMA Neurol 2015; 72(3): 287-94.
[http://dx.doi.org/10.1001/jamaneurol.2014.4144] [PMID: 25622185]

[19]   Lewczuk P, Matzen A, Blennow K, *et al.* Cerebrospinal fluid Abeta42/40 corresponds better tan Abeta42 to amyloid PET in Alzheimer's disease. J Alzheimers Dis 2017; 55(2): 813-22.
[http://dx.doi.org/10.3233/JAD-160722] [PMID: 27792012]

[20]   Bateman RJ, Xiong C, Benzinger TL, *et al.* Clinical and biomarker changes in dominantly inherited Alzheimer's disease. N Engl J Med 2012; 367(9): 795-804.
[http://dx.doi.org/10.1056/NEJMoa1202753] [PMID: 22784036]

[21]   Farrer LA, Cupples LA, Haines JL, *et al.* Effects of age, sex, and ethnicity on the association between apolipoprotein E genotype and Alzheimer disease. A meta-analysis. JAMA 1997; 278(16): 1349-56.
[http://dx.doi.org/10.1001/jama.1997.03550160069041] [PMID: 9343467]

[22]   Chouraki V, Seshadri S. Genetics of Alzheimer's disease. Adv Genet 2014; 87: 245-94.

[http://dx.doi.org/10.1016/B978-0-12-800149-3.00005-6] [PMID: 25311924]

[23]   Olsson B, Lautner R, Andreasson U, *et al.* CSF and blood biomarkers for the diagnosis of Alzheimer's disease: a systematic review and meta-analysis. Lancet Neurol 2016; 15(7): 673-84.
[http://dx.doi.org/10.1016/S1474-4422(16)00070-3] [PMID: 27068280]

[24] Blennow K, Mattsson N, Schöll M, Hansson O, Zetterberg H. Amyloid biomarkers in Alzheimer's disease. Trends Pharmacol Sci 2015; 36(5): 297-309.
[http://dx.doi.org/10.1016/j.tips.2015.03.002] [PMID: 25840462]

[25] Zetterberg H. Applying fluid biomarkers to Alzheimer's disease. Am J Physiol Cell Physiol 2017; 313(1): C3-C10.
[http://dx.doi.org/10.1152/ajpcell.00007.2017] [PMID: 28424166]

[26] Chhatwal JP, Schultz AP, Marshall GA, *et al.* Temporal T807 binding correlates with CSF tau and phospho-tau in normal elderly. Neurology 2016; 87(9): 920-6.
[http://dx.doi.org/10.1212/WNL.0000000000003050] [PMID: 27473132]

[27] Grahn A, Hagberg L, Nilsson S, Blennow K, Zetterberg H, Studahl M. Cerebrospinal fluid biomarkers in patients with varicella-zoster virus CNS infections. J Neurol 2013; 260(7): 1813-21.
[http://dx.doi.org/10.1007/s00415-013-6883-5] [PMID: 23471614]

[28] Kondziella D, Zetterberg H. Hyperphosphorylation of tau protein in superficial CNS siderosis. J Neurol Sci 2008; 273(1-2): 130-2.
[http://dx.doi.org/10.1016/j.jns.2008.06.009] [PMID: 18617192]

[29] Wallin AK, Blennow K, Zetterberg H, Londos E, Minthon L, Hansson O. CSF biomarkers predict a more malignant outcome in Alzheimer disease. Neurology 2010; 74(19): 1531-7.
[http://dx.doi.org/10.1212/WNL.0b013e3181dd4dd8] [PMID: 20458070]

[30] Tapiola T, Alafuzoff I, Herukka SK, *et al.* Cerebrospinal fluid beta-amyloid 42 and tau proteins as biomarkers of Alzheimer-type pathologic changes in the brain. Arch Neurol 2009; 66(3): 382-9.
[http://dx.doi.org/10.1001/archneurol.2008.596] [PMID: 19273758]

[31] Dumurgier J, Schraen S, Gabelle A, *et al.* Cerebrospinal fluid amyloid-b 42/40 ratio in clinical setting of memory centers: a multicentric study. Alzheimer's Res Ther 2015; 7: 1-9.

[32] Mattsson N, Insel PS, Landau S, *et al.* Diagnostic accuracy of CSF Ab42 and florbetapir PET for Alzheimer's disease. Ann Clin Transl Neurol 2014; 1(8): 534-43.
[http://dx.doi.org/10.1002/acn3.81] [PMID: 25356425]

[33] Jack CR Jr, Knopman DS, Jagust WJ, *et al.* Tracking pathophysiological processes in Alzheimer's disease: an updated hypothetical model of dynamic biomarkers. Lancet Neurol 2013; 12(2): 207-16.
[http://dx.doi.org/10.1016/S1474-4422(12)70291-0] [PMID: 23332364]

[34] Janelidze S, Zetterberg H, Mattsson N, *et al.* CSF Aβ42/Aβ40 and Aβ42/Aβ38 ratios: better diagnostic markers of Alzheimer disease. Ann Clin Transl Neurol 2016; 3(3): 154-65.
[http://dx.doi.org/10.1002/acn3.274] [PMID: 27042676]

[35] Simonsen AH, Herukka SK, Andreasen N, *et al.* Recommendations for CSF AD biomarkers in the diagnostic evaluation of dementia. Alzheimers Dement 2017; 13(3): 274-84.
[http://dx.doi.org/10.1016/j.jalz.2016.09.008] [PMID: 28341065]

[36] Zetterberg H. Plasma amyloid β-quo vadis? Neurobiol Aging 2015; 36(10): 2671-3.
[http://dx.doi.org/10.1016/j.neurobiolaging.2015.07.021] [PMID: 26234755]

[37] Kulstad JJ, Green PS, Cook DG, *et al.* Differential modulation of plasma beta-amyloid by insulin in patients with Alzheimer disease. Neurology 2006; 66(10): 1506-10.
[http://dx.doi.org/10.1212/01.wnl.0000216274.58185.09] [PMID: 16717209]

[38] Zetterberg H, Wilson D, Andreasson U, *et al.* Plasma tau levels in Alzheimer's disease. Alzheimers Res Ther 2013; 5(2): 9.
[http://dx.doi.org/10.1186/alzrt163] [PMID: 23551972]

[39] Shieh-Yueh Yang, Ming-Jang Chiu, Ta-Fu Chen, *et al.* Detection of Plasma Biomarkers Using Immunomagnetic Reduction: A Promising Method for the Early Diagnosis of Alzheimer's Disease Neurol Ther 2017; 6(Suppl 1): S37-56.

[40]   Bermejo-Pareja F, Antequera D, Vargas T, Molina JA, Carro E. Saliva levels of Abeta1-42 as potential biomarker of Alzheimer's disease: a pilot study. BMC Neurol 2010; 10: 108.
[http://dx.doi.org/10.1186/1471-2377-10-108] [PMID: 21047401]

[41]   Shi M, Sui YT, Peskind ER, *et al.* Salivary tau species are potential biomarkers of Alzheimer's disease. J Alzheimers Dis 2011; 27(2): 299-305.
[http://dx.doi.org/10.3233/JAD-2011-110731] [PMID: 21841250]

[42]   Gifford JL, Hunter HN, Vogel HJ. Lactoferricin: a lactoferrin-derived peptide with antimicrobial, antiviral, antitumor and immunological properties. Cell Mol Life Sci 2005; 62(22): 2588-98.
[http://dx.doi.org/10.1007/s00018-005-5373-z] [PMID: 16261252]

[43]   Welling MM, Nabuurs RJ, van der Weerd L. Potential role of antimicrobial peptides in the early onset of Alzheimer's disease. Alzheimers Dement 2015; 11(1): 51-7.
[http://dx.doi.org/10.1016/j.jalz.2013.12.020] [PMID: 24637300]

[44]   Carro E, Bartolomé F, Bermejo-Pareja F, *et al.* Early diagnosis of mild cognitive impairment and Alzheimer's disease based on salivary lactoferrin. Alzheimers Dement (Amst) 2017; 8: 131-8.
[http://dx.doi.org/10.1016/j.dadm.2017.04.002] [PMID: 28649597]

[45]   Wallin A, Blennow K, Fredman P, Gottfries CG, Karlsson I, Svennerholm L. Blood brain barrier function in vascular dementia. Acta Neurol Scand 1990; 81(4): 318-22.
[http://dx.doi.org/10.1111/j.1600-0404.1990.tb01562.x] [PMID: 2360399]

[46]   Zetterberg H. Neurofilament Light: A Dynamic Cross-Disease Fluid Biomarker for Neurodegeneration. Neuron 2016; 91(1): 1-3.
[http://dx.doi.org/10.1016/j.neuron.2016.06.030] [PMID: 27387643]

[47]   Blennow K. A Review of Fluid Biomarkers for Alzheimer's Disease: Moving from CSF to Blood. Neurol Ther 2017; 6 (Suppl. 1): 15-24.
[http://dx.doi.org/10.1007/s40120-017-0073-9] [PMID: 28733960]

[48]   Portelius E, Zetterberg H, Skillbäck T, *et al.* Cerebrospinal fluid neurogranin: relation to cognition and neurodegeneration in Alzheimer's disease. Brain 2015; 138(Pt 11): 3373-85.
[http://dx.doi.org/10.1093/brain/awv267] [PMID: 26373605]

[49]   Killiany RJ, Gomez-Isla T, Moss M, *et al.* Use of structural magnetic resonance imaging to predict who will get Alzheimer's disease. Ann Neurol 2000; 47(4): 430-9.
[http://dx.doi.org/10.1002/1531-8249(200004)47:4<430::AID-ANA5>3.0.CO;2-I] [PMID: 10762153]

[50]   Garibotto V, Herholz K, Boccardi M, *et al.* Clinical validity of brain fluorodeoxyglucose positron emission tomography as a biomarker for Alzheimer's disease in the context of a structured 5-phase development framework. Neurobiol Aging 2017; 52: 183-95.
[http://dx.doi.org/10.1016/j.neurobiolaging.2016.03.033] [PMID: 28317648]

[51]   Silverman DH, Small GW, Chang CY, *et al.* Positron emission tomography in evaluation of dementia: Regional brain metabolism and long-term outcome. JAMA 2001; 286(17): 2120-7.
[http://dx.doi.org/10.1001/jama.286.17.2120] [PMID: 11694153]

[52]   Klunk WE, Lopresti BJ, Ikonomovic MD, *et al.* Binding of the positron emission tomography tracer Pittsburgh compound-B reflects the amount of amyloid-beta in Alzheimer's disease brain but not in transgenic mouse brain. J Neurosci 2005; 25(46): 10598-606.
[http://dx.doi.org/10.1523/JNEUROSCI.2990-05.2005] [PMID: 16291932]

[53]   Wang Y, Klunk WE, Debnath ML, *et al.* Development of a PET/SPECT agent for amyloid imaging in Alzheimer's disease. J Mol Neurosci 2004; 24(1): 55-62.
[http://dx.doi.org/10.1385/JMN:24:1:055] [PMID: 15314250]

[54]   Nelson PT, Alafuzoff I, Bigio EH, *et al.* Correlation of Alzheimer disease neuropathologic changes with cognitive status: a review of the literature. J Neuropathol Exp Neurol 2012; 71(5): 362-81.
[http://dx.doi.org/10.1097/NEN.0b013e31825018f7] [PMID: 22487856]

[55] Schwarz AJ, Yu P, Miller BB, *et al.* Regional profiles of the candidate tau PET ligand 18F-AV-1451 recapitulate key features of Braak histopathological stages. Brain 2016; 139(Pt 5): 1539-50. [http://dx.doi.org/10.1093/brain/aww023] [PMID: 26936940]

[56] Wang L, Benzinger TL, Su Y, *et al.* Evaluation of tau imaging in staging Alzheimer disease and revealing interactions between beta-amyloid and tauopathy. JAMA Neurol 2016; 73(9): 1070-7. [http://dx.doi.org/10.1001/jamaneurol.2016.2078] [PMID: 27454922]

[57] Rubí S, Noguera A, Tarongí S, *et al.* Concordance between brain 18F-FDG PET and cerebrospinal fluid biomarkers in diagnosing Alzheimer's disease. Rev Esp Med Nucl Imagen Mol 2017; 20: S-2253-654X. [PMID: 28645685]

[58] Braak H, Thal DR, Ghebremedhin E, Del Tredici K. Stages of the pathologic process in Alzheimer disease: age categories from 1 to 100 years. J Neuropathol Exp Neurol 2011; 70(11): 960-9. [http://dx.doi.org/10.1097/NEN.0b013e318232a379] [PMID: 22002422]

[59] Thal DR, Beach TG, Zanette M, *et al.* [(18)F]flutemetamol amyloid positron emission tomography in preclinical and symptomatic Alzheimer's disease: specific detection of advanced phases of amyloid-β pathology. Alzheimers Dement 2015; 11(8): 975-85. [http://dx.doi.org/10.1016/j.jalz.2015.05.018] [PMID: 26141264]

[60] Rygiel K. Novel strategies for Alzheimer's disease treatment: An overview of anti-amyloid beta monoclonal antibodies. Indian J Pharmacol 2016; 48(6): 629-36. [http://dx.doi.org/10.4103/0253-7613.194867] [PMID: 28066098]

[61] Sevigny J, Chiao P, Bussière T, *et al.* The antibody aducanumab reduces Aβ plaques in Alzheimer's disease. Nature 2016; 537(7618): 50-6. [http://dx.doi.org/10.1038/nature19323] [PMID: 27582220]

[62] Jack CR Jr, Knopman DS, *et al.* Update on hypothetical model of Alzheimer's disease biomarkers. Lancet Neurol 2013; 12: 207-16. [http://dx.doi.org/10.1016/S1474-4422(12)70291-0] [PMID: 23332364]

[63] Sperling RA, Aisen PS, Beckett LA, *et al.* Toward defining the preclinical stages of Alzheimer's disease: recommendations from the National Institute on Aging-Alzheimer's Association workgroups on diagnostic guidelines for Alzheimer's disease. Alzheimers Dement 2011; 7(3): 280-92. [http://dx.doi.org/10.1016/j.jalz.2011.03.003] [PMID: 21514248]

[64] Butler D. Translational research: crossing the valley of death. Nature 2008; 453(7197): 840-2. [http://dx.doi.org/10.1038/453840a] [PMID: 18548043]

[65] Eckerström C, Olsson E, Bjerke M, *et al.* A combination of neuropsychological, neuroimaging, and cerebrospinal fluid markers predicts conversion from mild cognitive impairment to dementia. J Alzheimers Dis 2013; 36(3): 421-31. [http://dx.doi.org/10.3233/JAD-122440] [PMID: 23635408]

[66] Iaccarino L, Chiotis K, Alongi P, *et al.* A Cross-Validation of FDG- and Amyloid-PET Biomarkers in Mild Cognitive Impairment for the Risk Prediction to Dementia due to Alzheimer's Disease in a Clinical Setting. J Alzheimers Dis 2017; 59(2): 603-14. [http://dx.doi.org/10.3233/JAD-170158] [PMID: 28671117]

[67] Apostolova LG. Alzheimer Disease. Continuum (Minneap Minn) 2016; 22(2 Dementia): 419-34. [Minneap Minn]. [PMID: 27042902]

[68] Buchhave P, Minthon L, Zetterberg H, Wallin AK, Blennow K, Hansson O. Cerebrospinal fluid levels of β-amyloid 1-42, but not of tau, are fully changed already 5 to 10 years before the onset of Alzheimer dementia. Arch Gen Psychiatry 2012; 69(1): 98-106.

[http://dx.doi.org/10.1001/archgenpsychiatry.2011.155] [PMID: 22213792]

[69] Giovanni B Frisoni, Daniela Perani, Stefano Bastianello, *et al.* Biomarkers for the diagnosis of Alzheimer's disease in clinical practice: an Italian intersocietal roadmap. Neurobiology of Aging 2017; 52: 119-31.

[70] Jack CR Jr, Knopman DS, Jagust WJ, *et al.* Hypothetical model of dynamic biomarkers of the Alzheimer's pathological cascade. Lancet Neurol 2010; 9(1): 119-28.
[http://dx.doi.org/10.1016/S1474-4422(09)70299-6] [PMID: 20083042]

CHAPTER 6

Neuroimaging in Alzheimer's Disease

L. Díaz Rubia[1,*] and **J. García Verdejo[2]**

[1] *Department of Radiology, Hospital Clínico San Cecilio, Granada, Spain*
[2] *Service of Internal Medicine, General Hospital, Motril, Spain*

Abstract: Alzheimer's disease (AD) is a neurological degenerative disease that causes a progressive cognitive deterioration, being the main cause of dementia in elderly people at present. The diagnosis of Alzheimer's disease can be made with great precision through the use of clinical, neuropsychological and imaging evaluations, being of vital importance an early diagnosis to establish a treatment that improves the prognosis in these patients. From the neuroimaging point of view, magnetic resonance imaging (MRI) or computed tomography (CT) is recommended for the routine assessment of AD. MRI sequences in the coronal plane assess entorhinal and hippocampal cortical atrophy, typical at the onset of the disease. MRI volumetric sequences and subtraction are used in the evaluation of the progression of dementia. Positron emission tomography (PET) and single photon emission computed tomography (SPECT) are used to evaluate the prognosis of patients and in the differential diagnosis with other dementias. PET also serves to assess small visible alterations in very early stages, asymptomatic inclusions of the disease and in patients with predisposing genes to suffer AD.

Keywords: Alzheimer's disease(AD), neuroimaging, magnetic resonance imaging(MRI), computed tomography (CT), Positron emission tomography (PET), single photon emission CT (SPECT), brain atrophy, hippocampal atrophy, MRI Spectroscopy, Arterial Espin Labeling RM (ASL), Regional cerebral perfusion studies.

STRUCTURAL NEUROIMAGING IN ALZHEIMER'S DISEASE

TC and RMI

The anatomopathological changes in degenerative diseases of the central nervous system are related to brain atrophy which can be assessed by MRI. In the case of AD, the atrophy is more focused on the temporal lobe in its medial portion and in the hippocampus [1].

* Corresponding author L. Díaz Rubia: Department of Radiology, Hospital Clínico San Cecilio, Granada, Spain; Tel: 617496555; E-mail: laurix_dr@yahoo.es

The characteristic findings of AD are not readily apparent in the initial stages, in which there is a diffuse loss of cortical volume [2 - 4]. As the disease progresses, there is an accelerated loss of focal volume in the medial temporal lobes, particularly the hippocampus, the parahippocampal gyrus, the entorhinal cortex, and the amygdala. In clinical practice, the width of the lateral ventricle horn is the most reproducible measure to evaluate this atrophy. CT is a valid technique; usually is also the first test that is performed, especially if there are contraindications to the practice of MRI. With CT acquired in the orbitomeatal plane, the most adequate measure to distinguish the disease is the width of the lateral horn of the lateral ventricle. With these planes, a quotient of the radial width of the temporal horn with respect to the biparietal diameter is obtained. Thus, the volume loss is adjusted to cephalic diameter, being more useful for individual monitoring and intergroup differences. Normal subjects had a mean of 0.025, patients with AE of 0.038 and those with AD with extensive white matter lesions of 0.044 [5].

MRI Protocol in Alzheimer's Disease Study

T1-weighted sequences in the coronal plane are used for the evaluation of hippocampal atrophy (Fig. **1**).

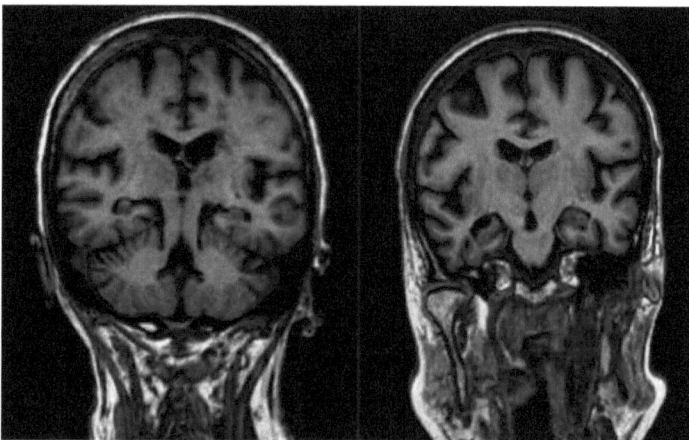

Fig. (1). Sequence weighted in T1 in the coronal plane of MRI of control patient (left) and patient with AD (right). The patient on the right shows atrophy of the right hippocampus. Department of Radiology, Hospital Clínico San Cecilio, Granada, Spain.

Some degenerative disorders are manifested by MRI signal alterations in midline structures that are visualized in sequences in the sagittal plane.

Other injuries such as infarcts, global cortical atrophy (GCA) and punctate white matter lesions are evaluated in FLAIR images and those lacunar infarcts that were not visualized will be studied in T2-weighted sequences, especially when they affect the thalamus or basal ganglia.

Signal falls in T2* images may be remnants of hemosiderin due to amyloid angiopathy but may also correspond to calcifications or iron deposits.

When neurodegenerative disorders with rapid onset are suspected, as in vasculitis, DWI images may be useful.

The MRI protocol to be followed in AD is summarized in Table **1**.

Table 1. RMI Protocol used in the AD.

Sag T1W	3D MPRAGE isotropic voxels coronal reformat perpendicular to hippocampi
Tra FLAIR	3 mm slices, 1mm istropic voxels
Tra T2W	3 mm slices, 1mm istropic voxels
Tra T2*	Gradient-echo, 3 mm slices, TE>20 ms, small flip angle

Neuropathological studies have shown that hippocampal volume with MRI is related to necropsy data. In a study to measure medial atrophy of the temporal lobe in RMI in AD, a sensitivity and specificity of 85% and 88%, respectively, were observed to detect the disease [6].

With MRI the best plane is the coronal and should always be evaluated at the same level (for example, mammillary bodies) to check its evolution. With a scale of only 5 degrees, adequate diagnostic accuracy can be achieved, ranging from 83% to 96% (Table **2**) [7].

Table 2. Criteria of Scheltens et al for the assessment of temporal lobe atrophy.

Grade	Choroidal Fissure Width	Temporal Horn Width	Hippocampus Height
0	Normal	Normal	Normal
1	mild increase	Normal	Normal
2	moderate increase	mild increase	mild decrease
3	severe increase	moderate increase	moderate decrease
4	severe increase	severe increase	severe decrease

Another potentially important application of MRI measurements is to serve as markers of worsening in patients with AD, and thus to be able to compare their evolution in patients treated with new therapies. For example, in a study of a muscarinic agonist, it was confirmed with brain MRI, obtained in 192 patients with one-year difference from the baseline study, that the deterioration was better seen in 99% of cases with measures of hippocampal atrophy than with cognitive or behavioral measures (p <0.001) [8]. This would reduce the sample for a clinical trial, such that while it would take 320 patients to detect a 50% reduction in the rate of worsening with the cognitive subscale score of the assessment of AD and 241 with the mini-mental test (MMSE), only 21 would be required if the hippocampus is measured and 54 if the lateral horn volume of the lateral ventricle is measured. The percentage of annual regional atrophy can be obtained with semiautomatic methods [9].

Scales Used in MRI to Assess Cerebral Atrophy

The GCA Scale

To measure global cortical atrophy, we use the GCA scale that is classified by degrees:

0: without atrophy

1: minimal or slight atrophy

2: atrophy is moderate

3: atrophy is important

This scale is not specific to Alzheimer's disease, but in this disease normally its values are high (Fig. **2**).

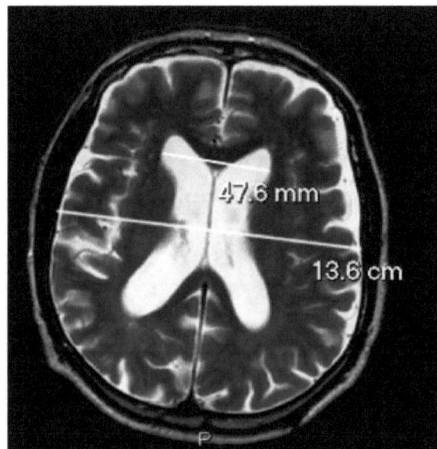

Fig. (2). Axial T2-weighted MRI scans showing cortical atrophy of bitemporal predominance with moderate dilatation of both lateral ventricles. Department of Radiology, Hospital Clínico San Cecilio, Granada, Spain.

Temporary Lobe Atrophy

It is measured with the MTA scale using T1-weighted sequences in the coronal plane performing the cortex at the hippocampal body level, considered abnormal in those over 75 years of age when the score is 3 or more points (2 may still be normal at this age)

The score is based on a visual score of the width of the choroidal fissure, the width of the temporal horn and the height of the formation of the hippocampus.

* 0: no atrophy
* 1: only widening of the choroidal fissure
* 2: also widening of the lateral horn of the lateral ventricle
* 3: moderate loss of hippocampal volume (decreased height)
* 4: severe loss of hippocampal volume

<75 years: 2 or more points are abnormal.
>75 years: 3 or more points are abnormal (Fig. **3**).

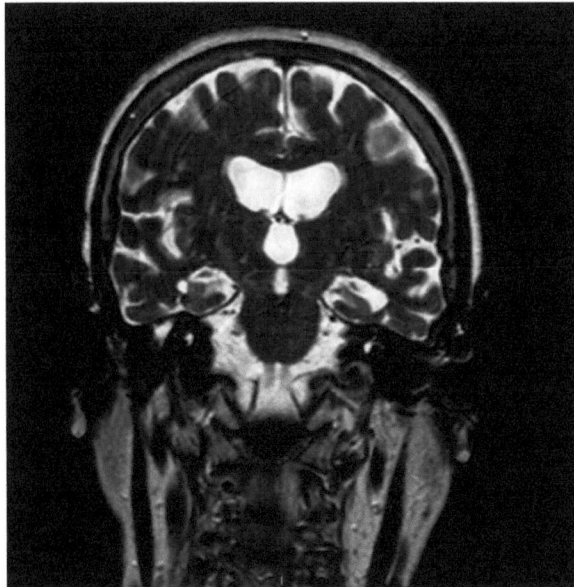

Fig. (3). Coronal T2-weighted MRI scans. Medial temporal lobe atrophy in AD. MTA=3. Department of Radiology, Hospital Clínico San Cecilio, Granada, Spain.

Patients with AD usually have a high score on the MTA scale but it is not a specific data of this disease. It is a very sensitive test, because if a patient with mild cognitive impairment (MCI) has a score in this low test, it will hardly evolve to AD [10]. AD is generally characterized by global atrophy with prominent atrophy of the medial temporal lobe. However, atypical forms of AD have been described with prominent posterior atrophy, especially frequent among patients with younger AD. This entity is also known as posterior cortical atrophy, but many studies have shown that AD pathology is most often present.

This absence of hippocampal atrophy is one of the thorny findings in AD that one can find.

MRI Images in Series

In addition to the existence of regional atrophy, another important structural imaging characteristic in AD is the progression of atrophy; we report an annual decrease in hippocampal volume approximately 2.5 times greater in patients with AD than in subjects of normal age and a relationship between memory loss and hippocampal damage across the spectrum from normal aging to dementia.

Neuroanatomical changes over time, in terms of atrophy of the temporal lobe or specifically of the hippocampus, may be too mild, different or topographically complex to detect them by visual inspection, or even with manual follow-up measures, as well as with voxel in the studio.

Vascular Changes

Late-onset AD is related to cerebrovascular disease and both can overlap, with mixed dementia then existing. In these patients hyperintense lesions of white matter and micro-bleeding will be observed in MRI.

The Fazekas scale provides an overall impression of the presence of white matter hyperintensities (WMH) throughout the brain. It is better scored on FLAIR or T2 cross-sectional images.

Fazekas score:

0: no injuries or few dotted

1: large number of dotted lesions

2: some injuries are confluent

3: large number of confluent lesions

Having 1 point on the Fazekas scale may be normal in elderly patients, while 2 or 3 points is always abnormal (Fig. **4**).

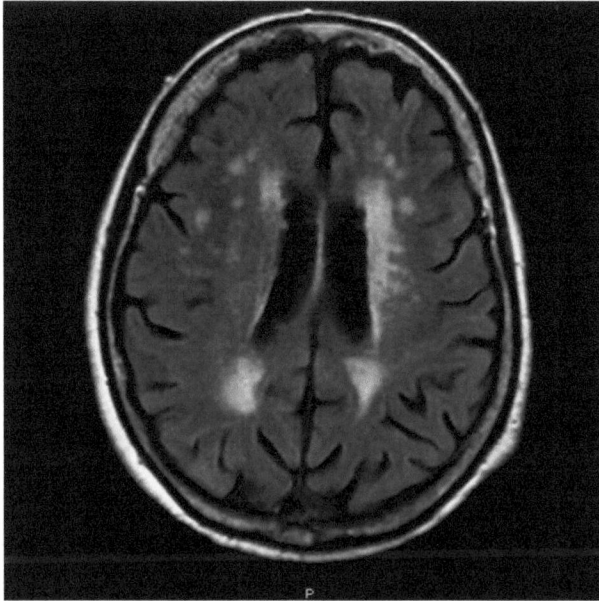

Fig. (4). FLAIR sequence in a patient with a large number of confluent white matter lesions (grade 3 of the Fazekas scale). Department of Radiology, Hospital Clínico San Cecilio, Granada, Spain.

In 600 elderly people, having 3 on the Fazekas scale predicted their intellectual disability within a year [11]. In another study in the follow-up period for 3 years, it was observed that those people who had a large number of hyperintense lesions of white matter suffered more cognitive deterioration than the rest [12].

With regard to WMH lesions, there is a correlation seen in some pre and postmortem MR studies [13]. However, leukoaraiosis is not visible macroscopically and there is no consensus in the literature on which technique is more sensitive in the detection of leukoaraiosis, whether MRI or biopsy [14]. Among the most common histopathological findings are loss of myelin and axons, astrogliosis, loss of oligodendrocytes, microglial activation and dilation of perivascular spaces.

FUNCTIONAL NEUROIMAGING IN ALZHEIMER'S DISEASE

MRI Spectroscopy (MRE)

As a complement to structural MRI, there is the possibility of using MRE, which is a noninvasive technique of neurochemical study of the brain in vivo, which makes a relative quantification of some chemical compounds that have a relevant role in brain function. Several studies have shown that the neuronal metabolite N-acetylaspartate (neuronal viability marker) decreases, suggesting neuronal destruction, in all cerebral hemispheres in patients affected by AD and the myoinositol component (glial activity and neurodegeneration) increases at the lobe level temporal and cingulate gyrus. This technique has a high sensitivity but low diagnostic specificity [15], comparing controls of patients with AD if the local concentration of NAA (N-acetylaspartate) and myoinositol by MRE is added to the measurement of hippocampal atrophy by structural MRI accuracy diagnosed up to 95% of these results accompanied by a clinical symptomatology of important neurological deterioration the MRE would guide towards the diagnosis of Alzheimer's disease [16].

Functional MRI Studies

Functional magnetic resonance imaging studies in patients with Alzheimer's have demonstrated hypo-activation of temporal lobe structures during memory tasks, while studies in the elderly with mild cognitive impairment (MCI) have reported an increase or decreased activation in the temporal lobe depending on the severity of cognitive impairment and underlying structural atrophy [17, 18]. In addition, recent findings of functional magnetic resonance imaging in patients with AD and MCI are beginning to reveal functional abnormalities between the temporal lobe and posteromedial regions such as the posterior cingulate cortex and precuneal cortex.

The most widely used functional magnetic resonance imaging technique to measure hemodynamic changes related to underlying cellular activity is based on the imaging of endogenous contrast in the blood that is oxygen-dependent (BOLD). Briefly, the relative decrease in the amount of deoxygenated hemoglobin improves the magnetic resonance signal locally in the brain areas activated during a particular cognitive task. In addition to the observed increases in the BOLD signal in areas of the activated brain, it has recently been shown that BOLD negative responses are also related to the underlying neuronal activity and have their origin in the decrease in neuronal activity below spontaneous activity in brain regions deactivated [19].

A recent study examined the brain network to investigate changes in connectivity between different regions using functional MRI at rest and using a mathematical algorithm, called graph theory, that allows quantifying the degree of correlation of the BOLD signal in a sample of voxels of the cerebral cortex [20]. The authors of the study have shown that by pattern recognition and brain network graphing using functional MRI at rest can help to diagnose AD [21].

Regional Cerebral Perfusion Studies with MRI

Regional perfusion can be assessed by brain MRI in several ways. Regional intravascular volume (rCBV) can be measured by rapid injection of a paramagnetic contrast that causes a decrease in microvessels. There are several studies of this type in AD [22, 23]. In a clinical study, Bozzao *et al* [24] found that the decrease in temporoparietal rCBV had a sensitivity of 90% to distinguish 16 patients with AD and mild cognitive impairment from 15 controls without any cognitive impairment and the specificity was of one 87%. The hippocampal cortex less clearly separated the patients (sensitivity 80% and specificity 65%).

This technique, which provides information similar to that provided by SPECT has, however, advantages:

1. Do not use ionizing radiation.

2. The quantification of regional cerebral flow is simpler.

3. Without moving the patient it can be registered with conventional MRI, with which the spatial resolution is better and infarcts or other ischemic alterations can be detected, frequent in elderly patients that, logically, influence the interpretation of the infusion alterations in AD.

On the other hand, compared with SPECT, this technique has a lower signal-to-noise ratio, is more sensitive to patient movement, and can lower blood flow if the transit time of blood from the base of the brain to tissue is greater than 1 second.

Arterial Spin Labeling RM (ASL)

ASL is a perfusion technique that can detect changes in brain function associated with AD in a manner similar to that obtained by a PET. ASL is potentially more suitable for the detection and follow-up of the disease since it is a non-invasive technique that does not require the use of radioisotopes or any contrast agent (the contrast is the protons of the blood in the blood) injected to the patient and is perfectly adapted to conventional MRI routines. ASL is proposed as a diagnostic alternative to PET, which in patients with AD and frontotemporal dementia reveals the same patterns of hypoperfusion as PET.

It was recently found that ASL is able to detect pathological areas found mainly in the parietal lobes and areas of the temporal cortex in patients with AD. Under suspicion of AD this perfusion technique can be used as a complement to structural MRI [25].

One study evaluated the potential of ASL for the diagnosis of AD and found that while the technique still offers suboptimal quality and limited brain coverage it may be able to delineate some known characteristics of the disease such as temporal lobe hypoperfusion. They also stressed that ASL has a great future for the individual diagnosis of AD because it does not use radiation or exogenous contrast media and allows repeated and reproducible measurements.

Diffusion Tensor image (DTI)

The DTI technique measures the movement of water molecules to characterize the microstructure of biological tissues and detect abnormalities of the white matter. In AD, damage to the cerebral cortex causes Wallerian involution with less fractional anisotropy at the predominantly temporal white matter level than groups of mild cognitive impairment or normal aging.

In a recent study, researchers evaluated the usefulness of this technique in patients with early onset Alzheimer's, primary progressive aphasia, and posterior cortical atrophy using MRI [26]. Thanks to this technique they were able to confirm that all groups show a pattern of white matter damage in the corpus callosum, cerebral fornix, anterior and posterior pathways as well as cortical atrophy in left temporoparietal and parietal regions. They also emphasized that the DTI technique has the potential to assess the extensive disruption of the brain network in AD even before the cognitive deficit is evident. Magnetic resonance plays a fundamental role in the diagnosis and monitoring of Alzheimer's disease, since it allows the study of the structure of the brain (loss of cerebral and hippocampal volume), cerebral perfusion(function), connectivity and brain activity a specific task). Although these techniques are currently in permanent use there is still a need for more extensive validation of each one of them.

Regional Cerebral Metabolism Studies with PET

Regional metabolism studies with PET have used 18F-2-deoxy-2-fluoro-D-glucose (FDG) as a metabolic marker.

Two clinical situations raised and continue to suggest the use of PET: DCL and atypical dementia, entities that PET can help to define.

As the degree of intensity of neuronal involvement in AD is marked more in the medial temporal region and in the cortex of parietal-temporal association, it is logical that these regions have a lower metabolism, since the synaptic density, which determines the regional metabolism, depends on the integrity not only of the efferent neuron, but also of the afferent neuron. The results of the neuropsychological tests should be interpreted with caution when trying to correctly define the cerebral location of the pathology.

Among the typical patterns of cortical hypometabolism in progressive degenerative dementia are (Fig. **5**):

1. Bilateral parietal temporal, by far the most frequent.

2. Bilateral Frontal.

3. Caudate the bilateral lenticular nucleus.

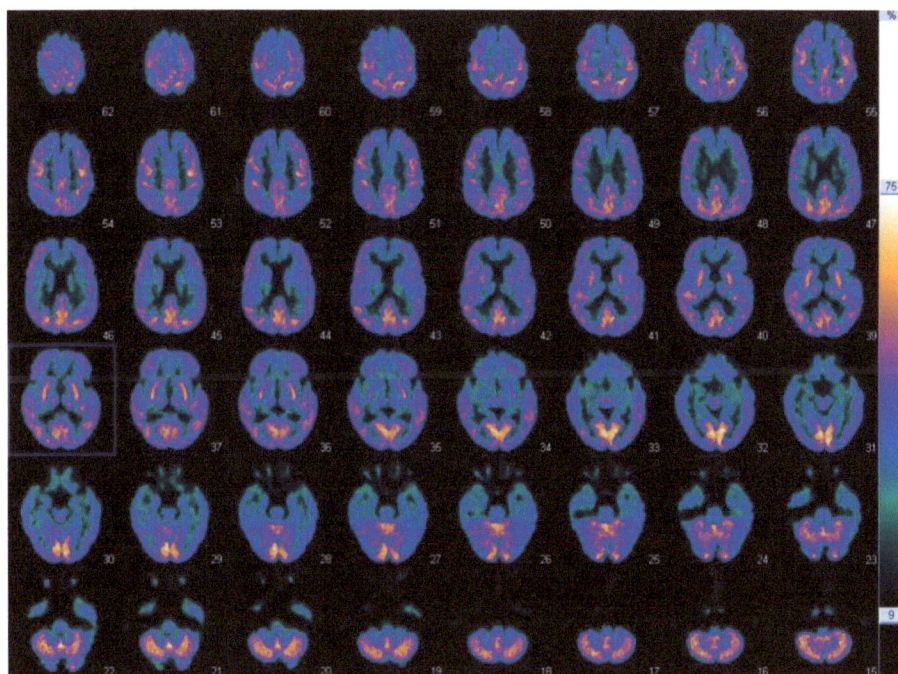

Fig. (5). FDG-PET study centered on posterior cingulate cortex and both frontal and temporal lobes. Nuclear Medicine Department, Hospital Clínico San Cecilio, Granada, Spain.

The major alterations occur in the association cortex, while the paracentral cortex and primary sensitivomotor areas are preserved.

Recently, using an automatic method of analysis of the voxel-based PET study (voxel-based morphometry), the distinction between healthy people and AD had a sensitivity of 93% and a specificity of 93%; even with mild dementia (with an MMSE $\geq$ 24), the sensitivity was still 84%, with a specificity of 93% [27]. An abnormal metabolism in people with MCI predicted a high risk of developing AD at two years.

Amyloid Deposition

Recently, a compound (FDDNP) has been developed which, in vitro, marks amyloid fibrils and tangles in the brains of patients with AD. In a pilot study with clinical PET in nine patients with AD and seven controls, this compound was more slowly removed from the brain of patients with AD [28]. Another compound that has already obtained PET images is PIB (Pittsburgh compound B), a derivative of thioflavin-T with high affinity for Abeta fibrils, which shows excellent entry into the brain and elimination of it [29]. In a study of 16 patients with incipient AD, deposits were detected in all but three patients and in none of the controls [30]. The distribution of deposits in the parietal-temporal and frontal cortex and posterior cingulate, being absent from the cerebellum, conforms to the regional distribution of amyloid deposits in AD known by conventional neuropathology.

Activation Studies with PET

PET was the first neuroimmune technique that allowed the obtaining of brain activation studies. For these studies, radioactive oxygen-labeled water ($H_2^{15}O$), a short half-life isotope, with which a temporal resolution of about 40 seconds is achieved. This isotope measures regional cerebral blood flow (rCBF). The regional flow increases at the same time as the regional oxygen demand due to a greater synaptic activity in this area of the brain. In these activation studies PET is performed at baseline and activation (for example, a person tries to remember something). The subtraction of the rCBF maps obtained in the two situations creates a map of the parts of the brain that are activated. They are compared with techniques such as parametric statistical mapping (SPM) [31].

Several studies of activation with $H_2^{15}O$ PET have shown that, in order to perform the same task, larger cortical areas are activated in people with AD or MCI than in healthy controls [32]. These findings have been interpreted as a compensatory mechanism cortically, where a greater extent of bark affected by AD has to be activated to achieve the same performance that healthy people achieve with activation of smaller areas.

Regional Cerebral Perfusion Sstudies with SPECT

The most commonly used tracers for studying brain perfusion with SPECT are technetium-labeled hexamethylpropyleneminoxime (99mTc-HMPAO) and technetium-labeled ethylcysteinate dimer (99mTc-ECD). There are many studies of SPECT in dementia of Alzheimer type [33] because it is easier to obtain a good study of SPECT than one of PET in patients with advanced dementia, so that the series of patients studied with SPECT usually contain more deteriorated patients. However, there are also several studies with SPECT in MCI and in pre-symptomatic individuals.

CONCLUDING REMARKS

Neuroimaging is already fundamental for the study and diagnosis of dementias. Its two aspects, both structural and functional neuroimaging, have experienced great progress in recent times, in addition to being more available today. Neuroimaging should be a diagnostic complement to clinical and analytical data.

The development of other techniques such as molecular diagnostics, including amyloid deposits, is occurring at such a high rate that the diagnosis of Alzheimer's disease is increasingly possible at earlier or even pre-symptomatic stages, which implies starting treatment earlier and, therefore, obtaining better results in the medium and long term in the morbidity and quality of life of these patients.

CONSENT FOR PUBLICATION

Not applicable.

CONFLICT OF INTEREST

None Declare

ACKNOWLEDGEMENT

None Declare

REFERENCES

[1]   Braak H, Braak E. Morphological criteria for the recognition of Alzheimer's disease and the distribution pattern of cortical changes related to this disorder. Neurobiol Aging 1994; 15(3): 355-6. [http://dx.doi.org/10.1016/0197-4580(94)90032-9] [PMID: 7936061]

[2]   Petrella JR, Coleman RE, Doraiswamy PM. Neuroimaging and early diagnosis of Alzheimer disease: a look to the future. Radiology 2003; 226(2): 315-36. [http://dx.doi.org/10.1148/radiol.2262011600] [PMID: 12563122]

[3]   Lehmann M, Koedam EL, Barnes J, *et al.* Posterior cerebral atrophy in the absence of medial temporal lobe atrophy in pathologically-confirmed Alzheimer's disease. Source Dementia Research Centre, UCL Institute of Neurology, Queen Square 2011.

[4]   Barnes J, Bartlett JW, van de Pol LA, *et al.* A meta-analysis of hippocampal atrophy rates in Alzheimer's disease. Neurobiol Aging 2009; 30(11): 1711-23. [http://dx.doi.org/10.1016/j.neurobiolaging.2008.01.010] [PMID: 18346820]

[5]   Zhang Y, Londos E, Minthon L, *et al.* Usefulness of computed tomography linear measurements in diagnosing Alzheimer's disease. Acta Radiol 2008; 49(1): 91-7. [http://dx.doi.org/10.1080/02841850701753706] [PMID: 18210318]

[6]   Scheltens P, Fox N, Barkhof F, De Carli C. Structural magnetic resonance imaging in the practical assessment of dementia: beyond exclusion. Lancet Neurol 2002; 1(1): 13-21. [http://dx.doi.org/10.1016/S1474-4422(02)00002-9] [PMID: 12849541]

[7]   Frisoni GB, Scheltens Ph, Galluzzi S, *et al.* Neuroimaging tools to rate regional atrophy, subcortical cerebrovascular disease, and regional cerebral blood flow and metabolism: consensus paper of the

EADC. J Neurol Neurosurg Psychiatry 2003; 74(10): 1371-81.
[http://dx.doi.org/10.1136/jnnp.74.10.1371] [PMID: 14570828]

[8]   Jack CR Jr, Slomkowski M, Gracon S, *et al.* MRI as a biomarker of disease progression in a therapeutic trial of milameline for AD. Neurology 2003; 60(2): 253-60.
[http://dx.doi.org/10.1212/01.WNL.0000042480.86872.03] [PMID: 12552040]

[9]   Thompson PM, Hayashi KM, de Zubicaray G, *et al.* Dynamics of gray matter loss in Alzheimer's disease. J Neurosci 2003; 23(3): 994-1005.
[http://dx.doi.org/10.1523/JNEUROSCI.23-03-00994.2003] [PMID: 12574429]

[10]   Burton EJ, Barber R, Mukaetova-Ladinska EB, *et al.* Medial temporal lobe atrophy on MRI differentiates Alzheimer's disease from dementia with Lewy bodies and vascular cognitive impairment: a prospective study with pathological verification of diagnosis. Brain 2009; 132(Pt 1): 195-203.
[http://dx.doi.org/10.1093/brain/awn298] [PMID: 19022858]

[11]   Inzitari D, Simoni M, Pracucci G, *et al.* Risk of rapid global functional decline in elderly patients with severe cerebral age-related white matter changes: the LADIS study. Arch Intern Med 2007; 167(1): 81-8.
[http://dx.doi.org/10.1001/archinte.167.1.81] [PMID: 17210882]

[12]   Inzitari D, Pracucci G, Poggesi A, *et al.* Changes in white matter as determinant of global functional decline in older independent outpatients: three year follow-up of LADIS (leukoaraiosis and disability) study cohort. BMJ 2009; 339: b2477.
[http://dx.doi.org/10.1136/bmj.b2477] [PMID: 19581317]

[13]   Grafton ST, Sumi SM, Stimac GK, Alvord EC Jr, Shaw CM, Nochlin D. Comparison of postmortem magnetic resonance imaging and neuropathologic findings in the cerebral white matter. Arch Neurol 1991; 48(3): 293-8.
[http://dx.doi.org/10.1001/archneur.1991.00530150061019] [PMID: 1705796]

[14]   Bronge L, Bogdanovic N, Wahlund LO. Postmortem MRI and histopathology of white matter changes in Alzheimer brains. A quantitative, comparative study. Dement Geriatr Cogn Disord 2002; 13(4): 205-12.
[http://dx.doi.org/10.1159/000057698] [PMID: 12006730]

[15]   Valenzuela MJ, Sachdev P. Magnetic resonance spectroscopy in AD. Neurology 2001; 56(5): 592-8.
[http://dx.doi.org/10.1212/WNL.56.5.592] [PMID: 11261442]

[16]   Schuff N, Capizzano AA, Du AT, *et al.* Selective reduction of N-acetylaspartate in medial temporal and parietal lobes in AD. Neurology 2002; 58(6): 928-35.
[http://dx.doi.org/10.1212/WNL.58.6.928] [PMID: 11914410]

[17]   Wagner AD. Early detection of Alzheimer's disease: an fMRI marker for people at risk? Nat Neurosci 2000; 3(10): 973-4.
[http://dx.doi.org/10.1038/79904] [PMID: 11017166]

[18]   Bookheimer SY, Strojwas MH, Cohen MS, *et al.* Patterns of brain activation in people at risk for Alzheimer's disease. N Engl J Med 2000; 343(7): 450-6.
[http://dx.doi.org/10.1056/NEJM200008173430701] [PMID: 10944562]

[19]   Johnson SC, Saykin AJ, Baxter LC, *et al.* The relationship between fMRI activation and cerebral atrophy: comparison of normal aging and alzheimer disease. Neuroimage 2000; 11(3): 179-87.
[http://dx.doi.org/10.1006/nimg.1999.0530] [PMID: 10694460]

[20]   Burggren AC, Small GW, Sabb FW, Bookheimer SY. Specificity of brain activation patterns in people at genetic risk for Alzheimer disease. Am J Geriatr Psychiatry 2002; 10(1): 44-51.
[http://dx.doi.org/10.1097/00019442-200201000-00006] [PMID: 11790634]

[21]   Minoshima S, Cross DJ, Foster NL, Henry TR, Kuhl DE. Discordance between traditional pathologic and energy metabolic changes in very early Alzheimer's disease. Pathophysiological implications.

Ann N Y Acad Sci 1999; 893: 350-2.
[http://dx.doi.org/10.1111/j.1749-6632.1999.tb07852.x] [PMID: 10672264]

[22]   González RG, Fischman AJ, Guimaraes AR, *et al.* Functional MR in the evaluation of dementia: correlation of abnormal dynamic cerebral blood volume measurements with changes in cerebral metabolism on positron emission tomography with fludeoxyglucose F 18. AJNR Am J Neuroradiol 1995; 16(9): 1763-70.
[PMID: 8693972]

[23]   Harris GJ, Lewis RF, Satlin A, *et al.* Dynamic susceptibility contrast MR imaging of regional cerebral blood volume in Alzheimer disease: a promising alternative to nuclear medicine. AJNR Am J Neuroradiol 1998; 19(9): 1727-32.
[PMID: 9802497]

[24]   Bozzao A, Floris R, Baviera ME, Apruzzese A, Simonetti G. Diffusion and perfusion MR imaging in cases of Alzheimer's disease: correlations with cortical atrophy and lesion load. AJNR Am J Neuroradiol 2001; 22(6): 1030-6.
[PMID: 11415893]

[25]   Du AT, Jahng GH, Hayasaka S, *et al.* Hypoperfusion in frontotemporal dementia and Alzheimer disease by arterial spin labeling MRI. Neurology 2006; 67(7): 1215-20.
[http://dx.doi.org/10.1212/01.wnl.0000238163.71349.78] [PMID: 17030755]

[26]   Teipel SJ, Grothe MJ, Filippi M, *et al.* Fractional anisotropy changes in Alzheimer's disease depend on the underlying fiber tract architecture: a multiparametric DTI study using joint independent component analysis. J Alzheimers Dis 2014; 41(1): 69-83.
[http://dx.doi.org/10.3233/JAD-131829] [PMID: 24577476]

[27]   Herholz K. PET studies in dementia. Ann Nucl Med 2003; 17(2): 79-89.
[http://dx.doi.org/10.1007/BF02988444] [PMID: 12790355]

[28]   Shoghi-Jadid K, Small GW, Agdeppa ED, *et al.* Localization of neurofibrillary tangles and beta-amyloid plaques in the brains of living patients with Alzheimer disease. Am J Geriatr Psychiatry 2002; 10(1): 24-35.
[http://dx.doi.org/10.1097/00019442-200201000-00004] [PMID: 11790632]

[29]   Klunk WE, Wang Y, Huang GF, *et al.* The binding of 2-(4'-methylaminophenyl)benzothiazole to postmortem brain homogenates is dominated by the amyloid component. J Neurosci 2003; 23(6): 2086-92.
[http://dx.doi.org/10.1523/JNEUROSCI.23-06-02086.2003] [PMID: 12657667]

[30]   Klunk WE, Engler H, Nordberg A, *et al.* Imaging brain amyloid in Alzheimer's disease with Pittsburgh Compound-B. Ann Neurol 2004; 55(3): 306-19.
[http://dx.doi.org/10.1002/ana.20009] [PMID: 14991808]

[31]   Ishii K, Willoch F, Minoshima S, *et al.* Statistical brain mapping of 18F-FDG PET in Alzheimer's disease: validation of anatomic standardization for atrophied brains. J Nucl Med 2001; 42(4): 548-57.
[PMID: 11337540]

[32]   Woodard JL, Grafton ST, Votaw JR, Green RC, Dobraski ME, Hoffman JM. Compensatory recruitment of neural resources during overt rehearsal of word lists in Alzheimer's disease. Neuropsychology 1998; 12(4): 491-504.
[http://dx.doi.org/10.1037/0894-4105.12.4.491] [PMID: 9805319]

[33]   Oukoloff K, Cieslikiewicz-Bouet M, Chao S, *et al.* PET and SPECT Radiotracers for Alzheimer's Disease. Curr Med Chem 2015; 22(28): 3278-304.
[http://dx.doi.org/10.2174/0929867322666150805094645] [PMID: 26242258]

CHAPTER 7

Palliative Care at the End of Life

Alfredo J. Pardo-Cabello[*]

Department of Internal Medicine. San Cecilio University Hospital, Granada, Spain

Abstract: In patients with advanced dementia, eating problems followed by infections were the most common complications. Several scales (NHO, ADEPT, PALIAR) have been proposed to estimate 6-months survival. In these patients, a better quality of life could be achieved with palliative care rather than with continued aggressive medical interventions. There is no evidence enough to suggest that enteral tube feeding is beneficial in these patients so careful hand feeding should be offered to them. There is a lack of randomized trials that had examined the effects of antibiotics both on survival and on symptom relief, so caution regarding the initiation of antimicrobial treatment in these patients is recommended. Pain is difficult to assess so it is frequently under-diagnosed and undertreated. No conclusive data are available to support the use of anti-dementia drugs in patients at stage 7 on the GDS scale. Palliative sedation is indicated in patients with advanced or terminal dementia that present a refractory suffering or symptoms. Midazolam is the first-line choice in palliative sedation in all prevailing symptoms, except delirium, in which case levomepromazine is the first-line choice. In dying patients, current medication should be assessed and non-essentials drugs should be discontinued. At the end of life, drugs needed to be continued should be switched to the subcutaneous route. If appropriate, a syringe driver may be used for continuous infusion. In dying patients, inappropriate interventions (*e.g.* intravenous fluids, antibiotics, blood tests, measurement of vital signs...) should be stopped.

Keywords: Alzheimer Disease, Anti-Bacterial Agents, Anti-Infective Agents, Aspiration Pneumonia, Decision Making, Deglutition Disorders, Dementia, Enteral Nutrition, Memantine, Mortality, Pain, Palliative Care, Palliative Sedation, Pressure Ulcer, Rivastigmine, Terminal Care, Vascular Dementia.

INTRODUCTION

Dementia constitutes a clinical syndrome characterized by a progressive impairment of one or more cognitive domains, producing a decline from the previous level of function to one that interferes with daily function and independence [1].

[*] **Corresponding author Alfredo J. Pardo-Cabello:** Department of Internal Medicine. San Cecilio University Hospital. Avda de la Investigación, s/n . 18016-Granada, Spain; Tel: +34 958.840.991; Fax: +34 958.122.307; E-mail: apardoc05@yahoo.es

Blas Gil-Extremera (Ed.)

Age has been reported by all epidemiological studies to be the main risk factor for dementia. Due to progressive ageing of the worldwide population, the overall burden associated with dementia is progressively increasing. Dementia has been estimated to affect 24 million people worldwide in 2001 and this number of patients was projected to almost double every 20 years [2].

In Europe, Lobo *et al* [3] reported an age-standardized prevalence of 6.4% for all kind of dementia in persons aged ≥65 years old, of which 4.4% was for Alzheimer Disease and 1.6% for vascular dementia; according to this study, the prevalence of dementia increased with age, ranging from 0.8% in the people aged 65-69 years to 28.5% in people aged 90 years and older. According to Sorbi *et al* [4], in the European Union, a crude prevalence of dementia was estimated at 6.2% what represents almost 9.95 million of patients with any form of dementia with an expectative of almost 14 million Europeans diagnosed with dementia in 2030.

CLINICAL COURSE AND END OF LIFE IN ADVANCED DEMENTIA

In relation to the clinical course of dementia, Mitchell *et al* [5] reported results after following 323 people with advanced dementia who lived in nursing homes in the United States of America. In this study [5], known as "Choices, Attitudes, and Strategies for Care of Advanced Dementia at the End-of-Life" (CASCADE), advanced dementia was considered if patient scored 5 or 6 on the Cognitive Performance Scale (CPS) [6] (a score of 5 in CPS equal to a score of 5.1±5.3 on the Mini-Mental State Examination) and a cognitive impairment due to dementia in stage 7 of the Global Deterioration Scale (GDS) [7]. Main results were [5]:

- 55% of residents died in the 18-months that lasted the study; the median survival was of 1.3 years.
- The eating problem was the most frequent clinical complication affecting 85.8% of patients followed by infections, mainly a febrile episode in 52.6% of patients and pneumonia in 41.1%.
- Other illnesses (*e.g.* hip fracture or myocardial infarction) were uncommon at the end of life.
- The adjusted 6-months mortality rate for patients with pneumonia was 46.7%; with a febrile episode, was 44.5% and with an eating problem, was 38.6%.
- In residents, the most common distressing symptoms were dyspnoea (46%) and pain (39.1%).
- 40.7% of residents underwent, at least, one burdensome medical intervention (including emergency room visit, hospitalization, tube feeding, or parenteral therapy) in their last 3 months of life.
- Residents with health care proxies who have an understanding of the clinical course and prognosis were likely to receive less aggressive interventions at the

end of life.

Among elderly people with advanced dementia, different criteria have been reported as prognostic indicators of mortality (Table **1**). In the United States, many efforts have been done in this issue because an estimated survival of six months or less is required to access to the US Medicare hospice benefit.

According to prognostic indicators included in Medicare hospice benefit guidelines [8] by National Hospice Organization (NHO), to be eligible for hospice (estimated survival of six months or less), patients with a diagnosis of dementia must meet both of the following requirements:

1. Stage 7 or higher on the Functional Assessment Staging (FAST) scale [9]: unable to walk, to dress or to bathe without assistance; intermittent or constant urinary and faecal incontinence; and no consistently meaningful verbal communication (the limitation of the ability to speak only six or fewer intelligible words or only stereotypical phrases).
2. Medical conditions: Patients must have presented, at least, one of the listed medical conditions over the last year:
    a. Aspiration pneumonia
    b. Septicaemia
    c. Pyelonephritis
    d. Recurrent fever treatment with antimicrobials
    e. Pressure ulcer, multiple, stage 3-4
    f. Dysphagia or refusal to eat of sufficient severity that patient cannot maintain sufficient fluid and calorie intake to sustain life with a weight loss of 10% in the last 6 months or a level of serum albumin below 2.5 g/dl.

The Advanced Dementia Prognostic Tool (ADEPT) is another model proposed to estimate survival in advanced dementia [10] and it is based on the sum of scores in twelve variables that best predicted survival in a study including 222,405 patients with advanced dementia who lived in nursing homes (Table **1**):

- Recent nursing home admission: 3.3 points
- Age: 60<75 years: 1 point; 70<75 years: 2 points; 75<80 years: 3 points; 80<85 years: 4 points; 85<90 years: 5 points; 90<95 years: 6 points; 95<100 years: 7 points; ≥100 years: 8 points.
- Sex: Male: 3.3 points.
- Pressure ulcers (at least one) in stage ≥ 2: 2.7 points.
- Dyspnoea: 2.7 points.
- Total functional dependence (Activity of Daily Living Score =28): 2.1 points.
- Bedfast most of day: 2.1 points.

- Faecal incontinence: 1.9 points.
- Body mass index < 18.5 kg/m^2: 1.8 points.
- Weight loss of > 5% of body weight in last 30 days, or > 10% in last 180 days: 1.6 points.
- Congestive heart failure: 1.5 points.

The area under Receiver Operating Characteristic (ROC) curve for the final model was 0.68 [10].

When ADEPT was compared to NHO hospice admission guidelines to estimate the 6-month survival in a cohort of 606 residents in nursing home with advanced dementia [11], the area under ROC for Medicare NHO guidelines was 0.55 (95% CI, 0.51-0.59), the specificity was 0.89 (95% CI, 0.86-0.92), and the sensitivity was 0.20 (95% CI, 0.13-0.28) while a cut-off of 13.5 points on the ADEPT score had a specificity of 0.89, an area under ROC of 0.58 (95% CI, 0.54-0.63) and a sensitivity of 0.27 (95% CI, 0.19-0.36).

On the other hand, among elderly people with advanced dementia, a systematic review of prognostic indicators of 6-month mortality published in 2013 reported that [12]:

- Seven studies were included after fulfilling criteria of inclusion: five were carried out in the United States and two in Israel.
- Among the studies, both methodology and prognostic outcomes showed a great variability.
- Six studies found that Functional Assessment Staging phase 7c, although currently used to assess hospice admission criteria in the United States, was not a reliable predictor of 6-month mortality.
- The most commonly identified prognostic variables were related to nutrition, or eating habits, followed by increased risk of dementia severity scales and comorbidities.
- Mitchell *et al* [16] reported that ADEPT scale had a moderate reliability as a prognostic indicator for 6-month mortality, with a good calibration, a high interrater reliability, and a high sensitivity (>90%), although low specificity (30%). Besides, Mitchell *et al* found the US Medicare hospice eligibility guidelines to have poor discrimination compared to the ADEPT scale.
- Further studies are needed to identify sensitive, reliable, and specific prognosticators that can be applied to the clinical setting and allow to increase the availability of palliative care to dementia patients.

Finally, PALIAR score was more recently (2014) developed and validated by Study Group of Polypathological Patient and Advanced Age of the Spanish

Society of Internal Medicine as a prognosticator of 6-month mortality in patients with advanced chronic medical conditions, including dementia [13]. This score is based on the sum of 6 partial scores [13]:

- Age ≥ 85 years: 3 points.
- Anorexia: 3.5 points.
- Functional class IV on Medical Research Council or New York Heart Association: 3.5 points.
- Presence of pressure ulcer(s): 3 points.
- Albumin <2.5 g/dl in laboratory parameter: 4 points.
- Eastern Cooperative Oncology Group Performance Status (ECOG-PS) ≥ 3 points: 4 points.

The area under the ROC curve for PALIAR score was 0.71 in the derivation cohort [13].

When PALIAR score was compared (Table **1**) to hospice admission guidelines [8] to estimate 6-month mortality in a validation cohort of 894 inpatients from Western areas of Spain [13], this new score showed higher sensitivity (85-90% *vs.* 69-75%, respectively) and negative predictive value (80-94% *vs.* 77-92%) than the National Hospice Organization criteria [8] in the low risk group (0 points); higher specificity (71-76% *vs.* 55-69% respectively) and positive predictive value (30-57% *vs.* 24-61% respectively) in the high-intermediate risk (≥ 4 points) and the highest risk group (≥ 7.5 points), with a specificity of 82-86% and a positive predictive value of 35-64% compared to aforementioned criteria [8].

In conclusion, although several scores have been proposed to estimate six-month survival in patients with advanced dementia, further studies are needed to identify reliable tools to be widely used in clinical settings.

Table 1. Models proposed to estimate 6-months survival in advanced dementia.

Model	Items Included	Sensitivity	Specificity	Area under ROC
NHO[A]	2	0.20	0.89	0.55
ADEPT[B]	12	0.27	0.89	0.58
PALIAR	6	0.85	0.86	0.69
[A] National Hospice Organization. [B]Advanced Dementia Prognostic Tool.				

PALLIATIVE CARE IN ADVANCED DEMENTIA

Definition of Palliative Care

World Health Organization (WHO) defined Palliative care as "an approach that improves the quality of life of patients and their relatives facing the problem associated with life-threatening illness, through the prevention and relief of suffering by early identification and faultless assessment and treatment of pain and other problems, physical, psychosocial and spiritual" [14].

Palliative care, according to WHO [14]:

- affirms life and consider death as a normal process;
- makes available relief from pain or other distressing symptoms;
- intends neither to accelerate or postpone death;
- offers a support system to help patients keeping as active as possible until death;
- integrates the spiritual and psychological aspects of patient care;
- helps the family cope during the patient's illness and in their own bereavement offering a support system;
- will improve the quality of life, and may also positively influence in the course of illness;
- is applicable early in the course of illness, added to other therapies that are intended to prolong life, such as chemotherapy or radiation therapy, and includes those research needed to better understand and manage distressing clinical complications;
- gives attention to the needs of patients and their families, using a team approach including bereavement counselling, if needed.

Palliative Care in Advanced Dementia

In patients with advanced dementia, a better quality of life could be achieved with palliative care rather than with continued aggressive medical interventions [5]. However, few studies have analyzed the impact of palliative care interventions in patients with advanced dementia.

A systematic review by Murphy *et al* [15] assessed the effect of palliative care in patients suffering advanced dementia and concluded that:

- Only two studies carried out in people with advanced dementia were identified focusing palliative care interventions.
- As blinding, logically, was not possible, both studies were at high risk of bias. Besides, the small sample sizes meant that the overall evidence was very low.

- Among patients with advanced dementia hospitalized for an acute illness, one randomized controlled trial including 99 participants found that a palliative care plan was more likely to be developed for participants in the intervention group (treated by palliative care team). However, while in hospital, the plan was only adopted for two participants included in the intervention group. On hospital discharge, the palliative care plan was more likely to be available in the intervention group. No evidence was found that the intervention affected in-hospital mortality, clinical care provided during admission, or decisions to abstain from cardiopulmonary resuscitation in the hospital.
- Other randomized controlled trial evaluated the effect of a decision aid giving written information to families of people with advanced dementia that explained the different methods that can be used to feed. Besides, intervention surrogates had lower scores for decisional conflict measured on the Decisional Conflict Scale and were more likely than participants in the control group to discuss feeding options with a clinician.
- Scarce high-quality studies have been finished regarding palliative care interventions in patients with advanced dementia. There is no evidence enough to assess the impact of the palliative care interventions in people with advanced dementia.
- Six studies in course at the time of the aforementioned systematic review show an increasing interest by researchers in this area.

Decision Making in Advanced Dementia

According to Mitchell [16], the planning of advance care is essential in the management of people with advanced dementia, and it is associated with avoiding unwanted or unnecessary treatments:

- Clinicians should educate to carers of patients about dementia evolution and expected clinical complications. If possible, patients should take part in the discussion about the care they wish to receive in advanced stages of illness.
- Establish written directives about patient preferences respect to receiving or not aggressive interventions, only treatment for comfort...
- When a target of care is established, consider interventions according to this goal.

Management of Specific Clinical Problems in Advanced Dementia

Eating Problems

As previously said, the most common complications in advanced dementia are eating problems [5]. The main causes of eating problems include oral dysphagia, pharyngeal dysphagia or refusal to eat. Dysphagia occurs independently of the aetiology of dementia and worsens along the clinical course of the neurodegenerative illness. Dysphagia is early onset especially in vascular dementia or in dementia associated with motor symptoms.

In cases of severe dysphagia, after ruling out or treating acute medical problems that can be associated with dysphagia, there are two options: long-term feeding tube (percutaneous endoscopic gastrostomy and nasogastric tube) or oral feeding by hand.

In relation to the use of long-term feeding tube in dementia, a systematic review published in 2009 [17] concluded that:

- No randomized clinical trials were identified. Seven observational controlled studies were included: six of them evaluated mortality and one assessed nutritional outcome.
- No evidence of increased survival was found in patients receiving enteral tube feeding.
- No studies examined the quality of life. No evidence of benefit in the prevalence of pressure ulcers or in terms of nutritional status was found.
- There is a lack of data on the adverse effects of this intervention.
- Insufficient evidence is available to suggest that enteral tube feeding is beneficial in patients with advanced dementia.

After this systematic review, a prospective study [18] published in 2012, and based on a cohort of 36,492 nursing home residents with advanced dementia, concluded that neither insertion of percutaneous endoscopic gastrostomy tubes nor the timing of insertion affects the survival of these patients.

On the other hand, a systematic review [19], published in 2011, analyzed the benefits of oral feeding options in people with dementia and reported that:

- The use of oral supplements in people with dementia was evaluated in thirteen controlled studies and assisted feeding or other interventions were assessed in twelve controlled trials.
- Trials provided a moderate evidence for the use of high-calorie supplements to promote weight gain in people with dementia, but a low evidence for the use of modified foods, appetite stimulants, and assisted feeding.
- No differences in terms of function or survival were found.
- Among people with dementia and feeding problems, high-calorie supplements and other oral feeding options can be useful to help them to increase weight; however, it is unlikely that they are able to improve other outcomes. These

supplements and other oral feeding options could be considered alone or in combination as an alternative to tube feeding.

After aforementioned studies, in 2014, the American Geriatrics Society published a position statement of about feeding tubes in advanced dementia [20]. This document states that [20]:

- Feeding tubes are not recommended for older adults with advanced dementia. As hand feeding has demonstrated to be as good as tube feeding in terms of survival, functional status, aspiration pneumonia, and comfort, careful hand feeding should be recommended. Besides, tube feeding has associated, in these patients, with agitation, healthcare use due to tube-related complications, greater use of chemical and physical restraints, and development of new decubitus ulcers.
- Tube feeding is a medical therapy. An individual's surrogate decision-maker can decline or accept this medical intervention according to prior stated wishes of the patient, what it is thought the individual would want, or the advance directives.
- Efforts to improve oral feeding by creating patient-centred approaches to feeding and altering the environment should be part of usual care for older adults with advanced dementia.
- To understand the previously stated wishes of the people (through review of advance directives and with surrogate caregivers) regarding tube feeding and to incorporate these wishes into the care plan is the responsibility of all health care members involved in caring for residents in long-term care settings.
- Institutions such as hospitals, nursing homes, and other care settings should not impose obligations or exert pressure on individuals or providers to institute tube feeding. They should promote choices, endorse shared and informed decision-making, and honor preferences regarding tube feeding.

Fever and Infections

An intercurrent infection should be ruled out in case of fever in patients with advanced dementia. Pneumonia and urinary tract infection are the most common causes of infection in these patients [5, 21]. The use of antibiotics is extensive in these patients [16]. In one prospective study [21] based on a cohort of 362 nursing home residents with severe dementia, 72.4% of the suspected infections were treated with antibiotics, but only 44% of them (19% in cases of urinary tract infections) had presented minimum clinical criteria supporting antimicrobial prescribing. The misuse in antimicrobial use constitutes an unnecessary treatment burden and increases multidrug-resistant organisms what is an emerging public health problem [16, 21].

In the CASCADE cohort, the residents with severe dementia and pneumonia who received any antibiotics improved their survival compared with no treatment patients but also had more discomfort than those who did not receive antimicrobials [22]. In this study, mortality rates were similar independently of the route of antimicrobial administration (oral, intramuscular, or intravenous) [22].

There is a lack of randomized studies that have analyzed the effects of antibiotics on survival or symptom relief in people with severe dementia [16]. Because of this, caution is recommended regarding the initiation of antimicrobial treatment in patients with advanced dementia [16]. In cases where comfort is the target, with a preference to forgo antibiotics, symptoms should be treated with only palliative measures [16]. In contrast, if prolongation of life is the goal, treatment with antibiotics is reasonable in case of there are clinical criteria to support it and if the treatment burden is minimized by using the least invasive route of administration and avoiding hospitalization, if possible [16].

Pain

As previously reported, in CASCADE cohort [5], pain (39.1%) was one of the most common distressing symptoms in residents with severe dementia. In many cases, pain assessment is difficult in these patients and, because of this, it is frequently under-diagnosed and under-treated in these patients, as previously reported [23].

Several tools to assess discomfort and pain in non-communicative patients with advanced dementia have been developed as PAINAD [24], Abbey [25], PACSLAC-II [26] or DOLOPLUS-2 [27]. However, further research is needed before they can be universally recommended.

When pain is diagnosed or suspected in patients with advanced dementia, geriatric management approaches and, standard palliative care are recommended to be applied [16].

Discontinuation of Anti-Dementia Drugs and other Chronic Medication

The use of chronic medications should coincide with the targets of care; so the drugs with doubtful clinical benefit should be stopped [16]. A cross-sectional study [28] based in the United States nationwide long-term care pharmacy database showed that:

• At least one medication with questionable benefit was prescribed to 54% of nursing home residents with advanced dementia.

- The most commonly prescribed drugs with questionable benefit were cholinesterase inhibitors (36%), memantine hydrochloride (25%), and lipid-lowering agents (22%).
- High facility-level use of feeding tubes increased the likelihood of receiving these drugs.
- The likelihood of receiving these drugs was reduced in residents who had a feeding tube, eating problems, a do-not-resuscitate order, or were enrolled in hospice.
- Among patients with severe dementia who were prescribed these medications, the costs of these drugs with questionable benefit accounted for 35.2% of the total average 90-day medication expenditures.

Besides, patients at stage 7 on the Global Deterioration Scale have not been included in clinical trials of the use of cholinesterase inhibitors and memantine; therefore, there are no compelling data to support the use of these drugs in patients with late-stage dementia [16].

Treatments to Avoid in Advanced Dementia

According to Spanish Clinical Practice Guidelines for dementia [29], in patients with severe dementia and in the terminal phase of life, extraordinary therapeutic procedures should be avoided because they are considered futile and may cause adverse effects and discomfort to patients.

As extraordinary therapeutic procedures are considered cardiopulmonary resuscitation, mechanical ventilation and hemodialysis because they have not demonstrated to reduce mortality or improve survival in this dementia stage [29].

Cardiopulmonary Resuscitation

In a study where 84 cognitively normal older adults were surveyed [30], about three-fourths of participants stated they would not want cardiopulmonary resuscitation, use of a ventilator, or intravenous or enteral tube feeding with the milder forms of dementia, and 95% or more of participants would not want these procedures with advanced dementia.

In people who are old or frail, cardiopulmonary resuscitation is commonly unsuccessful [31]. An overall likelihood of surviving discharge was 1 in 8 for patients who undergo cardiopulmonary resuscitation and 1 in 3 for patients who survive cardiopulmonary resuscitation according to a study [32] that analyzed rates of immediate survival and survival to discharge for adult patients undergoing in-hospital cardiopulmonary resuscitation; this study concluded that dementia was associated with failure to survive to discharge (OR 3.1; 95% CI 1.1, 8.8) [32].

Besides, cardiopulmonary resuscitation has demonstrated different rates of survival depending on where it is provided. In hospital settings, the patients most likely to survive cardiopulmonary resuscitation (30% survival to discharge) are the monitored ones who suffer ventricular tachyarrhythmias [33], but the overall rate of survival to discharge is about 16-17% [33, 34].

On the other hand, published data about outcomes from cardiopulmonary resuscitation in nursing homes are scarce [31]; data from studies carried out in the United States show a survival rate to hospital discharge of 0-5% [35, 36]. A study that analyzed the benefits of cardiopulmonary resuscitation in nursing home concluded that this procedure will benefit only a small percentage of nursing home patients who sustain cardiac arrest and suggested that cardiopulmonary resuscitation in nursing home only should be initiated when cardiac arrest is witnessed and it should only be continued in cases where initial documented cardiac rhythm is ventricular tachycardia or ventricular fibrillation [36].

In the UK, a joint statement from the Resuscitation Council (UK), the British Medical Association, and the Royal College of Nursing [37] considered that there is no benefit in cardiopulmonary resuscitation if the patient "will never have awareness or the ability to interact and is, therefore, unable to experience benefit".

In conclusion and according to recommendations of Spanish guidelines in dementia [29], cardiopulmonary resuscitation is not warranted in people with advanced dementia because it is an extraordinary therapeutic procedure that does not contribute a significant benefit.

Hemodialysis

Dementia is associated with a higher risk of mortality, hospitalizations, and withdrawal from hemodialysis [38]. A study based on a cohort of 16,694 patients in dialysis showed that, after adjustment for confounding factors, dementia was associated with an increased risk of dialysis withdrawal (RR 2.01, 95% confidence interval (CI) 1.57-2.57) and death (RR 1.48, 95% CI 1.32-1.66) [39].

Patients with dementia before hemodialysis initiation have been reported to have a 2-year survival of 24% compared to 66% for those without a diagnosis of dementia [40]; besides, this study showed an average survival for patients with dementia of 1.09 years *vs.* 2.7 years in patients without dementia with an adjusted hazard ratio of 1.87 (95% CI 1.77-1.98). The authors of the aforementioned study [40] concluded that patients with dementia should be considered for time-limited trials of dialysis and careful discussion in choosing whether to pursue initiation of dialysis or palliative care.

A recently published study [41] reported that patients with dementia had a higher risk of all-cause mortality in the first 6 months after dialysis initiation (adjusted hazard ratio, 1.25; 95% CI, 1.12-1.38) compared to patients without dementia.

In conclusion, in patients with severe dementia, dialysis is not recommended because it is not associated to benefit [29].

Palliative Sedation

A recently published systematic review [42] evaluated and compared systematically the palliative sedation guidelines among different countries and with the European Association for Palliative Care (EAPC) palliative sedation Framework. After analyzing a total of 13 guidelines, the authors of this review concluded that [42]:

- All guidelines defined palliative sedation in analogous ways, as an intervention only instituted for the purpose of refractory symptom control.
- All guidelines mentioned among the indications of palliative sedation that the 'suffering' should have been appropriately diagnosed and treatments for symptoms sought and tried, or at least carefully considered and found to be futile.
- Palliative sedation could be intermittent and temporary, or continuous until death. Besides, sedation could be deep (patient is asleep and unresponsive) or light (or superficial).
- Indications for using palliative sedation, the requirements for obtaining patient consent and direction for the actual administration, including dose titration, patient monitoring, and care were presented in all guidelines.
- The most common indicators were dyspnoea and terminal restlessness or delirium.
- On calculating the overall scores for developmental quality using the AGREE II instrument, nine guidelines were ranked moderate-high, and three were 'recommended for use', being they scored above 60% for the rigor of development.
- Guidelines from Spain [43], the Netherlands, and Japan were recommended for use in their current form because they satisfied the criteria for quality in the developmental process according to AGREE II criteria.

Definition of Palliative Sedation

According to Spanish Clinical Practice Guidelines for Palliative Care [43], palliative sedation is understood as the deliberate administration of drugs, in the dosage and combinations required to reduce the consciousness of a patient with an advanced or terminal illness, both when necessary to adequately alleviate one or more refractory symptoms and with their explicit consent.

Sedation in agony is a singular case of palliative sedation and it is defined as the deliberate administration of drugs to achieve alleviation of physical or psychological suffering, not attainable by other measures, through the sufficient deep and likely irreversible reduction of the consciousness of a patient whose death is foreseen to be very close [43].

Palliative Sedative Process in Agony

The palliative sedation process in agony has to satisfy a series of requirements [43, 44]:

- A correct therapeutic indication (existence of a refractory physical or psychic suffering or symptom at the end of patient's life) established by the doctor and, if possible, validated by another physician.
- Professionals with clear and complete information about the process, with a record on the medical history.
- The explicit consent of the patient, or the family if the patient is incompetent.
- Administration of the necessary doses and combinations of drugs to achieve the appropriate sedation level.

Therapeutic Indication

The correct prescription of palliative sedation requires [43]:

- Careful assessment of the diagnosis of end-of-life.
- Presence of refractory physical or psychic suffering and symptoms.
- Assessment of the patient's competence in decision-making [44].

End-of-Life Diagnosis (Terminality)

Apart from the medical prediction, the use of validated instruments to estimate the survival or functional state, such as the aforementioned NHO, ADEPT or PALIAR scores, may be useful as well as the presence of prognostic factors.

Refractory Suffering and Symptoms

A refractory symptom is understood as a suffering that cannot be appropriately controlled despite the efforts to find a tolerable treatment, which does not compromise consciousness and in a reasonable period of time [43].

A distinction between avoidable and non-avoidable suffering is crucial to determine on which aspects of avoidable suffering is possible (through symptom control, psychosocial interventions, care of the environment...) [43].

When the intervention possibilities run out, it is understood that the suffering is refractory [43]. In the case of uncertainty about the refractory nature of a symptom, consultation with other experts is recommended [44].

It is necessary to make sure that all intervention possibilities to control symptoms have been tried [43]. This is especially important in the case of pain [43]. Before deciding upon a sedation procedure, correct treatment of pain must be guaranteed [43].

Assessment of the Patient's Competence in Decision-Making

An assessment of the patient's competence is crucial [43]; in other words, his or her capacity to understand relevant information, express their wishes and know the implications and consequences of their decision [44].

The patient's competence should be appraised by an experienced team [43]. The involvement and coordination with the Primary Care physician is a key point at this point [43].

Patient's Consent

Consent means that the patient is competent to make decisions and that, adequately informed, expresses his/her explicit desire for sedation [43].

Competent Patient

Verbal consent is considered to be sufficient, although sometimes it could be given by writing [43]. A record must be always kept in the medical history [43].

Incompetent Patient

Firstly, the Preliminary Instructions and Living Wills Registry must be consulted [43]. If the patient has not left a written record of his/her wishes in relation to decisions at the end of life, the medical team must appraise the patient's wishes with family or friends' help, considering the previously expressed desires and values [43]. In this case, the communication process with family must satisfy the same requirements as necessary to obtain the patient's consent and which have been described before. In this case, sedation should be agreed with the family.

Due to the complexity of making decisions on sedation, when this situation is foreseeable, it is important to work with the patient regarding his opinion on this issue in advance and as a preventive measure, before agony arrives [43].

Therapeutic Privilege

If the patient has stated his/her will of not to be informed, this decision must be taken into account, determined by the therapeutic indication and with the express consent of the family [43].

Information to be Communicated

The medical team must determine and individually consider the benefits and possible harm of the information that will be disclosed [44], which will be comprised of the following data [43, 44]:

- Patient's situation: physical situation, incurability, expected survival.
- Suffering (presence of refractory suffering, causes of suffering, treatments that have been tested, the reasoning of the sedation decision).
- The objective of sedation (alleviate suffering).
- Sedation method: medication that reduces the level of consciousness with the option to discontinue sedation.
- Sedation effects: on the level of consciousness, communication, oral intake, the possibility of complications...
- Treatment and care after sedation, to maximize comfort.
- Expected results if sedation is not carried out: other alternatives, the degree of suffering, expected survival.

Health professionals must carefully consider the preferences of both patient and family, explaining to the family that their role is to estimate the patient's desire, that the family is not totally responsible for all the patient's decisions and that the team should share the responsibility of the decision of sedation [44].

Information to the Therapeutic Team

Professional involved in caring for the patient is advised to have a knowledge of the sedation process [43].

Drug Administration

There is little scientific evidence regarding what kind of medication and dosage must be used for palliative sedation [43 - 45].

A review on terminal sedation in palliative medicine based on thirteen series and fourteen case reports concluded that [45]:

- Three hundred and forty-two patients received eleven non-opioid drugs.
- Concurrent opioids were prescribed in most the patients.
- Terminal sedation was prescribed to most of the patients in an inpatient hospice unit.
- The most commonly used sedative was midazolam.
- The rate of good response, defined as an adequate sedation, ranged between 75% and 100%.
- The median survival after the initiation of terminal sedation was greater than 1 day.
- No agent appears to have superior efficacy than others or limiting toxicity.

The most commonly used drugs for sedation are benzodiazepines (midazolam), neuroleptics (levomepromazine), barbiturates (phenobarbital) and anaesthetics (propofol) [43].

Opioids are not recommended as a specific medication to induce palliative sedation, but they will be used concomitantly when the refractory symptom is pain or dyspnea or when the patient was taking them previously [43, 45].

Opioids should not be discontinued even when comfort is achieved because palliative sedation (using benzodiazepines, neuroleptics, barbiturates or anaesthetics) do not provide analgesia. Analgesia must be provided prior to and during use of palliative sedation with appropriate opioid and non-opioid options.

Midazolam

Midazolam is the most commonly employed sedation drug. Midazolam is the first-line choice if dyspnea, pain, bleeding, anxiety or panic are the prevailing symptoms [43]. It is available in ampules of 15 mg/3 ml. It can be used by subcutaneous (not included in the technical data sheet) or intravenous route [43]:

- Subcutaneous route:
  - Induction (bolus): 2.5 – 5 mg until sedation.
    Double dosage in case of patients that were already taking benzodiazepines.
  - Initial subcutaneous continuous infusion: 0.4 – 0.8 mg/h.
    Double dosage in case of patients that were already taking benzodiazepines.
  - Rescue (bolus): The same dosage as used in induction bolus (2.5 – 5 mg).

○ Maximum daily dosage: 160 – 200 mg per day.
- Intravenous route:
    ○ Induction (bolus): 1.5 – 3 mg / 5 minutes until sedation.
    ○ Initial intravenous continuous infusion: Total dosage needed to achieve induction x 6 / 24h (*e.g.* if 3 mg midazolam were needed to achieve sedation, the total dosage in intravenous continuous infusion is 3 x 6 = 18 mg midazolam/day).
    ○ Rescue (bolus): The same dosage as needed in induction.

Levomepromazine

Levomepromazine is a sedating antipsychotic used as the first-line choice for sedation if the prevailing symptom is delirium. It is available in ampules of 25 mg/1 ml. It can be used by subcutaneous (not included in the technical data sheet) or intravenous route [43]:

- Subcutaneous route:
    ○ Induction (bolus): 12.5 – 25 mg.
    ○ Initial subcutaneous continuous infusion: 100 mg/day.
    ○ Rescue (bolus): 12.5 mg.
    ○ Maximum daily dosage: 300 mg per day.
- Intravenous route:
    ○ Normally half the dosage by the subcutaneous route.

Propofol

Propofol is an ultra-rapid-acting general anaesthetic used as the second-line choice in cases of refractory agitation that have not responded to midazolam with/or levomepromazine in a hospital setting. The previous discontinuation of benzodiazepines perfusion or neuroleptics is needed in case of use of propofol. Besides, it is needed to reduce opioids to half dosage. It is available in vials and ampules of 10 mg in 1 ml and 20 mg in 1 ml. It can be only used by intravenous route and it is an in-hospital drug [43]:

- Intravenous route:
    ○ Induction (bolus): 1 – 1.5 mg/kg.
    ○ Initial intravenous continuous infusion: 2 mg/kg/h.
    ○ Rescue (bolus): Bolus of 50% the induction dosage.

After starting pharmacological sedation, the level of consciousness of patient should be monitored, using measures as Ramsay scale [46], and leaving a record of this on the medical history [43].

Ethical and Legal Considerations

The ethical and legal principles for sedation include [43, 44]:

- Appropriate indication and practice.
- Intentionality: the objective is to alleviate suffering.
- The principle of proportionality: considering the patient´s situation, the intensity of suffering, the absence of other palliative methods and the estimated survival, sedation is the most proportionate option among other therapeutic possibilities. It means reaching a balance between benefits (alleviation of suffering) and risks (reduction of the level of consciousness, the effect on survival).
- The principle of autonomy: in agreement to the applicable legislation, the patient owns the right to information and is entitled, after receiving adequate information, to freely decide between the available clinical options. The exceptions are therapeutic privilege (expressed desire of the patient to not be informed or total/almost total convincement that the information represents greater harm to the patient) and the situation of emergency (when there is an immediate serious risk to the physical or psychic integrity of the patient and it is not possible to obtain his/her authorization). Sedation requires delegated consent when the patient is not competent. It is always recommended to agree to decisions with the family, both if the patient is competent or not.

Furthermore, the team must decide on the amount of information to be given and how to give it. Information should be given about the voluntary nature of the sedation decision. The team should confirm that the decision of the patient is not affected by psychological or social pressure.

CARE OF THE DYING PATIENT

At the end of life of patients with advanced dementia, it is essential to "diagnose dying" in order to care for these patients [47]. Diagnosing dying is an important clinical skill. The key element in diagnosing dying is that the members of the multi-professional team caring for the patient agree that the patient is likely to die [47]. Once the team has diagnosed dying, the team can refocus care appropriately for the patient.

The goals of care for patients in the dying phase include [47]:

- Current medication assessed and non-essentials drugs should be stopped.
- Drugs that are needed to be carried on, such as opioids, anxiolytics, and antiemetic, should be switched to the subcutaneous route. If appropriate, a syringe driver may be used for continuous infusion.

- Subcutaneous drugs should be prescribed according to an agreed protocol (including those for pain and agitation) as required.
- Inappropriate medical interventions, including antibiotics, intravenous fluids or drugs, blood tests, and measurement of vital signs, should be stopped.
- Patients in the dying phase should not undergo "cardiopulmonary resuscitation", because this constitutes an inappropriate and futile medical intervention [47, 48].
- Clinical evolution of patient should be regularly followed up and good symptom control carried on, including control of pain and agitation.
- The patients' insight into their condition should be sensitively and appropriately assessed.
- The family's insight into the patient's condition should be assessed and issues related to dying and death explored sensitively and appropriately.
- The family should be told that the clinical expectation is that the patient is dying and will die.
- If families are told clearly that the patient is dying they have the opportunity to ask questions, say their goodbyes, stay with the patient, contact relevant people, and prepare themselves for the death.
- Contact telephone numbers should be given to relatives of patients dying in the community so that they have access to advise and help on a 24-hour basis.
- Sensitivity to the patient's religious, spiritual and cultural background is essential.
- In the dying phase, formal religious traditions may have to be observed and may influence the care of the body after death.
- Relatives should be dealt with in a compassionate manner after the patient's death.

CONSENT FOR PUBLICATION

Not applicable.

ACKNOWLEDGEMENTS

Declared none

CONFLICT OF INTEREST

The author confirms that this chapter contents have no conflict of interest.

REFERENCES

[1]   Diagnostic and Statistical Manual of Mental Disorders. Fifth Edition (DSM-5)., Arlington: American Psychiatric Association 2013.

[2]   Ferri CP, Prince M, Brayne C, *et al.* Global prevalence of dementia: a Delphi consensus study. Lancet 2005; 366(9503): 2112-7.
[http://dx.doi.org/10.1016/S0140-6736(05)67889-0] [PMID: 16360788]

[3]   Lobo A, Launer LJ, Fratiglioni L, *et al.* Prevalence of dementia and major subtypes in Europe: A collaborative study of population-based cohorts. Neurology 2000; 54(11) (Suppl. 5): S4-9.
[PMID: 10854354]

[4]   Sorbi S, Hort J, Erkinjuntti T, *et al.* EFNS-ENS Guidelines on the diagnosis and management of disorders associated with dementia. Eur J Neurol 2012; 19(9): 1159-79.
[http://dx.doi.org/10.1111/j.1468-1331.2012.03784.x] [PMID: 22891773]

[5]   Mitchell SL, Teno JM, Kiely DK, *et al.* The clinical course of advanced dementia. N Engl J Med 2009; 361(16): 1529-38.
[http://dx.doi.org/10.1056/NEJMoa0902234] [PMID: 19828530]

[6]   Morris JN, Fries BE, Mehr DR, *et al.* MDS Cognitive Performance Scale. J Gerontol 1994; 49(4): M174-82.
[http://dx.doi.org/10.1093/geronj/49.4.M174] [PMID: 8014392]

[7]   Reisberg B, Ferris SH, de Leon MJ, Crook T. The Global Deterioration Scale for assessment of primary degenerative dementia. Am J Psychiatry 1982; 139(9): 1136-9.
[http://dx.doi.org/10.1176/ajp.139.9.1136] [PMID: 7114305]

[8]   Medical guidelines for determining prognosis in selected non-cancer diseases. Hosp J 1996; 11(2): 47-63.
[http://dx.doi.org/10.1080/0742-969X.1996.11882820] [PMID: 8949013]

[9]   Reisberg B. Functional assessment staging (FAST). Psychopharmacol Bull 1988; 24(4): 653-9.
[PMID: 3249767]

[10]   Mitchell SL, Miller SC, Teno JM, Davis RB, Shaffer ML. The advanced dementia prognostic tool: a risk score to estimate survival in nursing home residents with advanced dementia. J Pain Symptom Manage 2010; 40(5): 639-51.
[http://dx.doi.org/10.1016/j.jpainsymman.2010.02.014] [PMID: 20621437]

[11]   Mitchell SL, Miller SC, Teno JM, Kiely DK, Davis RB, Shaffer ML. Prediction of 6-month survival of nursing home residents with advanced dementia using ADEPT *vs* hospice eligibility guidelines. JAMA 2010; 304(17): 1929-35.
[http://dx.doi.org/10.1001/jama.2010.1572] [PMID: 21045099]

[12]   Meghan A. Brown, Elizabeth L Sampson, Louise Jones, and Anna M Barron. Prognostic indicators of 6-month mortality in elderly people with advanced dementia: A systematic review. Palliat Med 2013; 27: 389-400.
[http://dx.doi.org/10.1177/0269216312465649] [PMID: 23175514]

[13]   Bernabeu-Wittel M, Murcia-Zaragoza J, Hernández-Quiles C, *et al.* Development of a six-month prognostic index in patients with advanced chronic medical conditions: the PALIAR score. J Pain Symptom Manage 2014; 47(3): 551-65.
[http://dx.doi.org/10.1016/j.jpainsymman.2013.04.011] [PMID: 23998780]

[14]   World Health Organization. WHO definition of palliative care [Accessed 2017-09-02]; Available at: http://www.who.int/ cancer/palliative/definition/en/

[15]   Murphy E, Froggatt K, Connolly S, *et al.* Palliative care interventions in advanced dementia. Cochrane Database Syst Rev 2016; 12: CD011513.
[PMID: 27911489]

[16]   Mitchell SL. Clinical Practice. Advanced Dementia. N Engl J Med 2015; 372(26): 2533-40.
[http://dx.doi.org/10.1056/NEJMcp1412652] [PMID: 26107053]

[17]   Sampson EL, Candy B, Jones L. Enteral tube feeding for older people with advanced dementia. Cochrane Database Syst Rev 2009; 15(2): CD007209.

[PMID: 19370678]

[18]   Teno JM, Gozalo PL, Mitchell SL, *et al.* Does feeding tube insertion and its timing improve survival? J Am Geriatr Soc 2012; 60(10): 1918-21.
[http://dx.doi.org/10.1111/j.1532-5415.2012.04148.x] [PMID: 23002947]

[19]   Hanson LC, Ersek M, Gilliam R, Carey TS. Oral feeding options for people with dementia: a systematic review. J Am Geriatr Soc 2011; 59(3): 463-72.
[http://dx.doi.org/10.1111/j.1532-5415.2011.03320.x] [PMID: 21391936]

[20]   American Geriatrics Society feeding tubes in advanced dementia position statement. J Am Geriatr Soc 2014; 62(8): 1590-3.
[http://dx.doi.org/10.1111/jgs.12924] [PMID: 25039796]

[21]   Mitchell SL, Shaffer ML, Loeb MB, *et al.* Infection management and multidrug-resistant organisms in nursing home residents with advanced dementia. JAMA Intern Med 2014; 174(10): 1660-7.
[http://dx.doi.org/10.1001/jamainternmed.2014.3918] [PMID: 25133863]

[22]   Givens JL, Jones RN, Shaffer ML, Kiely DK, Mitchell SL. Survival and comfort after treatment of pneumonia in advanced dementia. Arch Intern Med 2010; 170(13): 1102-7.
[http://dx.doi.org/10.1001/archinternmed.2010.181] [PMID: 20625013]

[23]   Nygaard HA, Jarland M. Are nursing home patients with dementia diagnosis at increased risk for inadequate pain treatment? Int J Geriatr Psychiatry 2005; 20(8): 730-7.
[http://dx.doi.org/10.1002/gps.1350] [PMID: 16035124]

[24]   Warden V, Hurley AC, Volicer L. Development and psychometric evaluation of the Pain Assessment in Advanced Dementia (PAINAD) scale. J Am Med Dir Assoc 2003; 4(1): 9-15.
[http://dx.doi.org/10.1097/01.JAM.0000043422.31640.F7] [PMID: 12807591]

[25]   Abbey J, Piller N, De Bellis A, *et al.* The Abbey pain scale: a 1-minute numerical indicator for people with end-stage dementia. Int J Palliat Nurs 2004; 10(1): 6-13.
[http://dx.doi.org/10.12968/ijpn.2004.10.1.12013] [PMID: 14966439]

[26]   Chan S, Hadjistavropoulos T, Williams J, Lints-Martindale A. Evidence-based development and initial validation of the pain assessment checklist for seniors with limited ability to communicate-II (PACSLAC-II). Clin J Pain 2014; 30(9): 816-24.
[http://dx.doi.org/10.1097/AJP.0000000000000039] [PMID: 24281294]

[27]   Lefebvre-Chapiro S. The Doloplus-2 scale - evaluating pain in the elderly. Eur J Palliat Care 2001; 8: 191-4.

[28]   Tjia J, Briesacher BA, Peterson D, Liu Q, Andrade SE, Mitchell SL. Use of medications of questionable benefit in advanced dementia. JAMA Intern Med 2014; 174(11): 1763-71.
[http://dx.doi.org/10.1001/jamainternmed.2014.4103] [PMID: 25201279]

[29]   Grupo de trabajo de la Guía de Práctica Clínica sobre la atención integral a las personas con enfermedad de Alzheimer y otras demencias. Guía de Práctica Clínica sobre la atención integral a las personas con enfermedad de Alzheimer y otras demencias. Plan de Calidad para el Sistema Nacional de Salud del Ministerio de Sanidad, Política Social e Igualdad. Agència d'Informació, Avaluació i Qualitat en Salut de Cataluña; 2010. Guías de Práctica Clínica en el SNS: AIAQS Núm. 2009/07.

[30]   Gjerdingen DK, Neff JA, Wang M, Chaloner K. Older persons' opinions about life-sustaining procedures in the face of dementia. Arch Fam Med 1999; 8(5): 421-5.
[http://dx.doi.org/10.1001/archfami.8.5.421] [PMID: 10500515]

[31]   Conroy SP, Luxton T, Dingwall R, Harwood RH, Gladman JR. Cardiopulmonary resuscitation in continuing care settings: time for a rethink? BMJ 2006; 332(7539): 479-82.
[http://dx.doi.org/10.1136/bmj.332.7539.479] [PMID: 16497767]

[32]   Ebell MH, Becker LA, Barry HC, Hagen M. Survival after in-hospital cardiopulmonary resuscitation. A meta-analysis. J Gen Intern Med 1998; 13(12): 805-16.
[http://dx.doi.org/10.1046/j.1525-1497.1998.00244.x] [PMID: 9844078]

[33]   Peberdy MA, Kaye W, Ornato JP, *et al.* Cardiopulmonary resuscitation of adults in the hospital: a report of 14720 cardiac arrests from the National Registry of Cardiopulmonary Resuscitation. Resuscitation 2003; 58(3): 297-308.
[http://dx.doi.org/10.1016/S0300-9572(03)00215-6] [PMID: 12969608]

[34]   Ballew KA, Philbrick JT, Caven DE, Schorling JB. Predictors of survival following in-hospital cardiopulmonary resuscitation. A moving target. Arch Intern Med 1994; 154(21): 2426-32.
[http://dx.doi.org/10.1001/archinte.1994.00420210060007] [PMID: 7979838]

[35]   Benkendorf R, Swor RA, Jackson R, Rivera-Rivera EJ, Demrick A. Outcomes of cardiac arrest in the nursing home: destiny or futility? [see comment]. Prehosp Emerg Care 1997; 1(2): 68-72.
[http://dx.doi.org/10.1080/10903129708958790] [PMID: 9709340]

[36]   Tresch DD, Neahring JM, Duthie EH, Mark DH, Kartes SK, Aufderheide TP. Outcomes of cardiopulmonary resuscitation in nursing homes: can we predict who will benefit? 1993; 95(2): 123-30.
[http://dx.doi.org/10.1016/0002-9343(93)90252-K]

[37]   Decisions Relating to Cardiopulmonary Resuscitation: a joint statement from the British Medical Association, the Resuscitation Council (UK) and the Royal College of Nursing. J Med Ethics 2001; 27(5): 310-6.
[http://dx.doi.org/10.1136/jme.27.5.310] [PMID: 11579186]

[38]   Anand S, Kurella Tamura M, Chertow GM. The elderly patients on hemodialysis. Minerva Urol Nefrol 2010; 62(1): 87-101.
[PMID: 20424572]

[39]   Kurella M, Mapes DL, Port FK, Chertow GM. Correlates and outcomes of dementia among dialysis patients: the Dialysis Outcomes and Practice Patterns Study. Nephrol Dial Transplant 2006; 21(9): 2543-8.
[http://dx.doi.org/10.1093/ndt/gfl275] [PMID: 16751655]

[40]   Rakowski DA, Caillard S, Agodoa LY, Abbott KC. Dementia as a predictor of mortality in dialysis patients. Clin J Am Soc Nephrol 2006; 1(5): 1000-5.
[http://dx.doi.org/10.2215/CJN.00470705] [PMID: 17699319]

[41]   Molnar MZ, Sumida K, Gaipov A, *et al.* Pre-ESRD Dementia and Post-ESRD Mortality in a Large Cohort of Incident Dialysis Patients. Dement Geriatr Cogn Disord 2017; 43(5-6): 281-93.
[http://dx.doi.org/10.1159/000471761] [PMID: 28448971]

[42]   Abarshi E, Rietjens J, Robijn L, *et al.* International variations in clinical practice guidelines for palliative sedation: a systematic review. BMJ Support Palliat Care 2017; 7(3): 223-9.
[PMID: 28432090]

[43]   Health Technologies Assessment Agency of the Basque Country. Madrid: National Plan for the NHS of the MSC. 2008. Clinical Practice Guidelines in the Spanish NHS: OSTEBA No. 2006/08.

[44]   Morita T, Bito S, Kurihara Y, Uchitomi Y. Development of a clinical guideline for palliative sedation therapy using the Delphi method. J Palliat Med 2005; 8(4): 716-29.
[http://dx.doi.org/10.1089/jpm.2005.8.716] [PMID: 16128645]

[45]   Cowan JD, Walsh D. Terminal sedation in palliative medicine--definition and review of the literature. Support Care Cancer 2001; 9(6): 403-7.
[http://dx.doi.org/10.1007/s005200100235] [PMID: 11585266]

[46]   Ramsay MA, Savege TM, Simpson BR, Goodwin R. Controlled sedation with alphaxalone-alphadolone. BMJ 1974; 2(5920): 656-9.

[http://dx.doi.org/10.1136/bmj.2.5920.656] [PMID: 4835444]

[47]   Ellershaw J, Ward C. Care of the dying patient: the last hours or days of life. BMJ 2003; 326(7379): 30-4.
[http://dx.doi.org/10.1136/bmj.326.7379.30] [PMID: 12511460]

[48]   Joint Working Party between the National Council for Hospice and Specialist Palliative Care Services and the Ethics Committee of the Association for Palliative Medicine of Great Britain and Ireland Ethical decision making in palliative care: cardiopulmonary resuscitation for people who are terminally ill. London: National Council for Hospice and Specialist Palliative Care Services 2002.

CHAPTER 8

Nutrition and Alzheimer's Disease

Cristina Fernández-García[*]

Cognitive Impairment Unit, Neurology Service, La Moraleja University Hospital, Madrid, Spain

Abstract: The pathophysiology of Alzheimer's disease is complex. Both genetic and environmental factors are considered to be involved. Among the latter, nutrition may play a major role. Longitudinal cohort studies have found that people who closely follow the Mediterranean diet, the DASH diet, and the MIND diet undergo less cognitive decline over time and have lower rates of dementia and Alzheimer's disease. However, interventional studies are needed to establish a causal relationship. In this connection, clinical studies based on the Mediterranean diet have reported positive results for cognitive performance. The beneficial results obtained by certain diets have not been achieved by supplementation with individual nutrients, suggesting that added benefit may be derived through the association of foodstuffs, for instance as occurs in the diet, as opposed to when they are administered separately. Research into nutrients beneficial to brain function has been carried out, and medical foods with good safety and tolerability profiles have been designed and have yielded promising results in the treatment of mild Alzheimer's disease.

Keywords: Alzheimer Disease, Mediterranean Diet, Nutrition, Prevention.

INTRODUCTION

A series of changes takes place in the brains of patients with Alzheimer's disease (AD), *e.g.*, the build-up of β-amyloid plaques, the formation of neurofibrillary tangles, neuron loss, and synaptic loss [1 - 4]. These changes in the brain are presumed to occur many years before cognitive function begins to deteriorate [5].

Until just a few years ago, diagnostic criteria for AD depended on the presence of a dementia syndrome [6, 7]. However, this can be regarded as the final stage of years of ongoing pathophysiological damage occurring in the brains of persons with AD, starting with a decline in certain cognitive functions (in general, significant impairment of episodic memory) and subsequently the onset of difficulty in performing the activities of daily living and fulfilment of the criteria for dementia [5]. A range of diagnostic criteria have thus been established to help

---

[*] **Corresponding author Cristina Fernández-García:**; Cognitive Impairment Unit, Neurology Service, La Moraleja University Hospital, Madrid, Spain; Tel: +34 91 7679237; E-mail: cfernandezg@sanitas.es

Blas Gil-Extremera (Ed.)

clinicians in their daily practice. First, the patient's cognitive status needs to be assessed. That is, cognitive decline that does not affect the activities of daily living represents mild cognitive impairment [8, 9], also termed mild neurocognitive disorder in the Diagnostic and Statistical Manual of Mental Disorders, Fifth Edition (DSM-5) [10]. By contrast, a patient who presents both cognitive impairment and difficulty in going about the activities of daily living unassisted receives a diagnosis of dementia [11] or major neurocognitive disorder (DSM-5) [10]. This is followed by an etiological diagnosis, most commonly AD [10, 12]. The diagnostic criteria for AD have lately been revised by several working groups [10, 13 - 16]; they all have in common the possible use of biomarkers without needing to fulfil the criteria for dementia.

AD becomes more frequent with advancing age [12, 17]. The figures reported in the World Alzheimer Report 2015 by Alzheimer's Disease International (ADI) furnish an idea of the extent of the problem, and it is estimated that the number of cases of dementia diagnosed will double every 20 years [17]. The number of people suffering from dementia worldwide was estimated at 46.8 million in 2015 and is expected to reach 74.7 million by 2030 and 131.5 million by 2050 [17]. Cases of cognitive impairment that do not fulfil the criteria for dementia also need to be taken into account. According to Plassman and colleagues, 5.4 million people in the United States have some type of cognitive impairment without dementia [18]. With progressive aging of the population, cognitive impairment and dementia can readily be seen to pose an extremely serious health threat [17, 18].

The various pathophysiological changes taking place in AD are considered to have multiple causes and to be conditioned by genetic and environmental factors [12]. The scientific evidence published to date suggests the existence of various risk factors for the onset of AD, some of which can be modulated, *e.g.*, hypertension during middle age, diabetes mellitus, smoking, depression, and a low level of education [19 - 21]. Conversely, a high level of education, regular physical and mental exercise, and a healthy diet may exert protective effects [19, 21].

Unfortunately, as yet there is no cure for AD; therefore, all actions aimed at preventing, or more precisely, delaying, the onset of disease symptoms and/or slowing disease progression when symptoms have appeared take on special importance. In 2014, ADI reported that delaying symptom onset for an average of five years could have the effect of lowering the total number of cases worldwide by 50% [19]. The Rotterdam Study raised the possibility of preventing onset of dementia in a substantial number of cases by removing the main modifiable risk factors [22].

Nutrition is one of the environmental factors that may play a major role in AD. Current evidence on its possible role in preventing AD is based on cross-sectional, cohort, and longitudinal studies and some clinical trials [23].

A useful starting point could be the data published by the IANA Task Force on Nutrition and Cognitive Decline with Aging, a collection of epidemiological studies suggesting that certain macro and micronutrients might exert a preventive effect on cognitive decline and dementia, though the data are not solid. Particular interest has centred on certain diets, such as the Mediterranean diet [23].

This article presents a review of the most significant evidence, focusing on the prevention of AD on the one hand and on therapeutic aspects on the other. Some studies have reported on the association between certain diets, certain macro and micronutrients, and cognitive impairment generally and AD in particular, and seek to identify modifiable risk/protective factors and thereby to undertake preventive steps [23].

There is a large volume of information. We will first look at the information currently available on the effects of certain diets consumed by the population on a daily basis on cognitive performance and on the onset of cognitive decline as well as on dementia syndrome in general and AD in particular. We will also examine the evidence currently available concerning the possible preventive effect of certain nutrients. Lastly, we will discuss nutrition and AD from a therapeutic standpoint.

DIET AND PREVENTION OF ALZHEIMER'S DISEASE

Our diet is one of the fundamental aspects of our lives. A number of articles have been published in recent years dealing with the association between ingesting certain nutrients and developing cognitive decline and dementia. What is more, the world's various populations combine foodstuffs in ways that gradually take hold as dietary patterns. The effect of a given nutrient may possibly not be the same when it is eaten on its own as when it is eaten in combination with other foodstuffs in the diet. Thus, assessing the behaviour of dietary patterns in specific populations over time holds particular interest; accordingly, we will look at the results of longitudinal cohort studies and interventional studies.

Mediterranean Diet

The Mediterranean diet has been a subject of interest in recent years because of the beneficial health effects reported by various studies [23]. It features consumption of fish, vegetables, legumes, fruits, grains, and unsaturated fatty acids, with olive oil being the main source of fat. Intake of dairy products, meat, and saturated fatty acids is low, and the diet also includes regular moderate intake of red wine [23]. The first aspect that should be noted is that the method used to assess the diet has itself been the subject of study. Most studies use the Mediterranean Diet Score (MedDietS) [24, 25].

Trichopoulou and colleagues used a semi-quantitative food frequency questionnaire to study the diets of 91 men and 91 women older than 70 years of age in three Greek populations (190 foods and beverages in all) [24]. They found eight features that characterized the Mediterranean diet: a proportionately high intake of monounsaturated as opposed to saturated fats, moderate consumption of alcohol, high consumption of legumes, high consumption of cereal grains (including bread and potatoes), high consumption of fruits, high consumption of vegetables, low consumption of meat and meat products, and low consumption of milk products [24]. The median sex-specific consumption of each food group was taken as the cut-off. The study concluded that the more the diet adhered to these features, *i.e.*, the higher the score, the lower the risk of death (a decrease of 17% for a one-point increase and of more than 50% for a four-point increase) [24].

In 2003, Trichopoulou and colleagues [25] published the results of a prospective longitudinal study of 22,043 adults ranging in age from 20 to 86 years in Greece. Using a semi-quantitative food frequency questionnaire, they identified 150 foods in 14 food groups [potatoes, vegetables, legumes, fruits and nuts, dairy products, cereals, meat, fish, eggs, monounsaturated lipids (mainly olive oil), poly-unsaturated lipids (vegetable-seed oils), saturated lipids and margarines, sugar and sweets, and non-alcoholic beverages]. The MedDietS was assessed on a scale ranging from 0 to 9. Median intake of each food group was calculated by sex, yielding a reference value (the higher the value, the greater the adherence to the diet). For beneficial foods like vegetables, legumes, fruits and nuts, cereals, and fish, a value of 0 was assigned if intake was below the cut-off, a value of 1 if it was above the cut-off. By contrast, for foods regarded as not affording health benefits (meat, poultry, and dairy products), intake above the median was assigned a value of 0 and intake below the median a value of 1. For alcohol, a value of 1 was assigned if intake was within a specified range. For the fat intake, the ratio of monounsaturated lipids to saturated lipids was used. Greater adherence to the diet was associated with a reduction in total mortality [the adjusted hazard ratio for death associated with a two-point increase in the MedDietS was 0.75 (95% confidence interval: 0.64 to 0.87)]. On assessing mortality from specific causes, the findings were the same for coronary heart disease [adjusted hazard ratio 0.67 (95% confidence interval: 0.47 to 0.94)] and for cancer [adjusted hazard ratio 0.76 (95% confidence interval: 0.59 to 0.98)].

In 2007, Panagiotakos and colleagues published a MedDietS on a scale ranging from 0 to 55 [26], calculated based on a self-administered food frequency questionnaire. As in the case of the MedDietS study by Trichopoulou and colleagues [25], intake of certain specified products was evaluated for a total of 11 food groups in all. Whole grain cereals, vegetables, fruits, legumes, potatoes, fish, and olive oil were considered beneficial. By contrast, meat and meat products, poultry, and milk products were regarded as non-beneficial. Each group was assigned a score of from 0 to 5. A total score of 0 was the lowest possible adherence to the Mediterranean diet, 55 the highest.

Looking at longitudinal cohort studies, the following studies that have tried to relate better cognitive performance to adherence to the Mediterranean diet are discussed below.

In the ILIDA study, Psaltopoulou and colleagues studied a cohort of 732 men and women 60 years of age or older who were residents of a region of Greece and took part in the EPIC–Greece (European Prospective Investigation into Cancer and Nutrition) cohort [27]. Participants were followed for between 6 and 13 years. A series of variables relating to diet and lifestyle habits were recorded on enrolment, but no cognitive evaluation was performed. The only assessment performed during the follow-up period was a Mini Mental State Examination (MMSE), and this is one of the study's limitations. The MedDietS was used, on a scale of from 0 to 9 [24, 25]. The study concluded that there was a non-significant weak positive association between the MMSE score and adherence to the Mediterranean diet [27]. In contrast, in a prospective study also carried out in a country in the Mediterranean region published in 2009, Feart and colleagues found evidence of a positive association between adherence to the Mediterranean diet and better cognitive performance, though no association with the onset of dementia [28]. The cohort of the Three-City study included 1,410 participants 65 years of age or older from the population of Bordeaux (France) who were re-examined at least once over the course of five years. Again the MedDietS was used, on a scale of from 0 to 9 [24, 25]. Neuropsychological evaluation at baseline and at follow-up included the MMSE and other neuropsychological tests to assess verbal fluency, immediate visual memory, and episodic verbal memory. Greater adherence to the Mediterranean diet was associated with a smaller decrease in the MMSE score but not with the other cognitive test results. Greater adherence to the Mediterranean diet was not associated with a risk of dementia onset [28].

Another large cohort study in a United States population reported similar results. The Chicago Health and Aging Project (CHAP) began in 1993 and included 6,158 subjects aged 65 years or more with follow-up every three years that included neuropsychological testing and other evaluations [29]. A subset of the total cohort that included those subjects who had undergone at least two neuropsychological evaluations was chosen and comprised 3,790 participants. The MedDietS was used, on a scale of from 0 to 55 [26]. The neuropsychological evaluation consisted of four tests, including the MMSE. After an average of 7.6 years of follow-up, an association between adherence to the Mediterranean diet and less cognitive decline was found. Another dietary pattern was also assessed for that same population, namely, the Healthy Eating Index–2005 (HEI-2005) based on the recommendations set out in the 2005 Dietary Guidelines for Americans [30]. That pattern shares some similarities with the Mediterranean diet (both recommend eating whole grain cereals, fruits, and vegetables), but there are also some differences, *e.g.*, the HEI-2005 does not have separate food groups for fish, poultry, alcohol (at least for its beneficial component), legumes, or nuts. At the end of the follow-up indicated above, no evidence of a positive association was found between adherence to the HEI-2005 and cognitive performance [29].

A number of articles of this same kind have been published online since 2012, reflecting a growing interest in the possible connection between the Mediterranean diet and better cognitive performance. Longitudinal studies of variable duration that included neuropsychological evaluation have relied on a range of different tests, and their findings have not all been concordant. Some have reported a positive association [31 - 38], while others have found no evidence of any such association [39 - 44].

Two studies stand out from among those reporting a positive association between the Mediterranean diet and better cognitive performance owing to their extended follow-up. One was the Supplementation with Vitamins and Mineral Antioxidants.2 (SU.VI.MAX.2) study carried out in France on 3,083 participants from the SU.VI.MAX study, with follow-up for 13 years, which concluded that a low MedDietS was significantly associated with lower test scores, but only for certain tests and not for global cognitive function. This study was subject to a limitation that should be noted, namely, no baseline neuropsychological evaluation was performed [31]. The Cache County Study on Memory, Health, and Aging in the United States is another study with longer than usual follow-up [34]. It had 3,831 subjects 65 years of age or older and concluded that participants having a higher MedDietS at baseline and over 11 years of follow-up also had a significantly higher score on the neuropsychological evaluation test used [Modified Mini-Mental State Examination (3MS)].

As already mentioned, some longitudinal studies have found no positive association between adherence to the Mediterranean diet and cognitive performance. Except for the report by Psaltopoulou and colleagues [27], conducted in Greece as discussed, the rest all took place outside the

Mediterranean region. Chief among these is the Australian cohort included in the PATH Through Life study [39], a prospective study carried out on 1,528 cognitively normal persons aged between 50 and 64 years. They were tested twice, four years apart, using the International Consensus Criteria, impairment on the Clinical Dementia Rating scale (Clinical Dementia Rating: 0.5) for cognitive assessment. The study concluded that there was no evidence that the Mediterranean diet protected against cognitive decline. It is important to note that the participants were younger than those included in other studies, who were mostly 65 years of age or older. Follow-up was not particularly long, and the study did not use a battery of neuropsychological tests or a test to evaluate global cognitive performance. Other studies that also did not find a positive association were carried out in the United States and were performed only on women [41 - 44].

In view of the above-mentioned results, there would appear to be conflicting data on the association between the Mediterranean diet and better cognitive performance. Studies that reported a positive association were likely to have a longer follow-up period and more comprehensive neuropsychological testing, so future studies should be structured along those lines.

Other studies have attempted to compile more precise results by focusing on the risk of suffering cognitive impairment, dementia, or AD.

In 2006, Scarmeas and colleagues published the results of follow-up of a multiethnic cohort in New York that included participants in two related cohorts recruited in 1992 (WHICAP 1992) and 1999 (WHICAP 1999) [45]. The association between adherence to the Mediterranean diet and the risk of suffering AD was examined in 2,258 participants without dementia recruited from the community and followed for four years, with evaluations every 1.5 years. Here again the MedDietS was used, on a scale of from 0 to 9 [24, 25]. At the starting and follow-up evaluations each subject underwent a medical examination and a battery of neuropsychological tests. Based on all the information compiled, neurologists and neuropsychologists diagnosed the presence or absence of dementia by consensus using the criteria of the Diagnostic and Statistical Manual of Mental Disorders, Revised Third Edition (DSM-III-R), with an etiological diagnosis where dementia was present (the criteria of the National Institute of Neurological and Communicative Disorders and Stroke-Alzheimer's Disease and Related Disorders Association were used to make the diagnosis of AD). Greater adherence to the Mediterranean diet was related to a lower risk of developing AD (hazard ratio: 0.91; 95% confidence interval: $0.83 - 0.98$; $p = 0.015$). The greater the adherence to the Mediterranean diet, *i.e.*, the higher the MedDietS, the lower the risk of AD, which is suggestive of a dose-response effect. The same findings were obtained when the analysis was adjusted for such potential confounding variables for AD as age, sex, ethnic group, educational level, APOE genotype, calorie intake, and body mass index. Diagnoses of AD took into account only diagnoses of cases of probable AD where the results were not affected by the concomitant presence of stroke. It should also be noted that there were no significant differences in the MedDietS of patients who were lost to follow-up and those who completed the study, as well as the MedDietS stability over the course of follow-up [45].

A subsequent study of 1,393 cognitively normal subjects also recruited from the two above-mentioned related cohorts (WHICAP I 1992) and (WHICAP II 1999) found that greater adherence to the Mediterranean diet was associated with a lower risk of developing cognitive impairment (the association being greater the higher the MedDietS, such that for the top tertile the hazard ratio was 0.72; 95% CI: 0.52 – 1.00; p = 0.05) [46]. Conversion to AD was also studied in those participants who had undergone cognitive decline, and the risk was found to be lower in those who adhered more closely to the Mediterranean diet (for the top-tertile MedDietS, the hazard ratio was 0.52; 95% CI: 0.30 – 0.91; p = 0.02) [46].

Gu and colleagues later studied 1,219 subjects aged 65 or older without dementia from the WHICAP II cohort. After a four-year follow-up the top tertile of adherence to the Mediterranean diet had a significantly lower probability (34%) of developing AD compared with the lowest tertile of adherence [47].

A Swedish cohort study carried out as part of the Uppsala longitudinal study of adult men used a modified MedDietS with a scale similar to the 0 to 9 MedDietS scale used by Trichopoulou and colleagues *et al.* [24, 25], except it did not include nuts. Follow-up was 12 years, and the Mediterranean diet was not associated with a lesser risk of AD (hazard ratio: 1.00; 95-% CI: 0.75-1.33) [48].

More recently, Wu and colleagues published a systematic literature review and meta-analysis and identified nine prospective studies [49]. Cluster analysis showed that compared with the category with the lowest Mediterranean diet score, the category with the highest Mediterranean diet score was inversely related to the development of cognitive disorders (mild cognitive impairment, dementia, or AD, depending on the study). In contrast, the category with the median score had no significant association with the incidence and risk of cognitive disorders. Dose-response analysis demonstrated a trend towards a linear relationship with the Mediterranean diet [49].

Observational longitudinal studies provide relevant data on the possible association between the Mediterranean diet and AD but no information on causality. In other words, the existence of that positive association does not mean that greater adherence as such is necessarily the cause. For this, interventional studies are indispensable.

The PREDIMED randomized primary cardiovascular risk prevention trial was carried out across multiple health centres in Spain [50]. Two versions of the Mediterranean diet, one supplemented with extra virgin olive oil (EVOO) and the other supplemented with mixed nuts, were tested on a population at high risk of cardiovascular disease against the low-fat diet customarily recommended to high-risk populations for primary prevention of cardiovascular disease. Martínez-Lapiscina and colleagues studied 522 participants at one of the participating centres (PREDIMED-NAVARRA) [50]. Participants were tested using the MMSE [51] and the clock-drawing test [52] 6.5 years after the intervention. The study found that intervention based on the Mediterranean diet enhanced by EVOO or nuts appeared to improve cognition compared with the low-fat diet, given that, after adjusting for various variables (including vascular risk factors), the Mediterranean diet + EVOO and the Mediterranean diet + nuts achieved significantly higher MMSE and clock-drawing test scores than the low-fat diet control group [50].

Valls-Pedret and colleagues analyzed another PREDIMED study subcohort (Barcelona-North PREDIMED) [53]. A full neuropsychological examination [Mini-Mental State Examination, Rey Auditory Verbal Learning Test (RAVLT), Animal Semantic Fluency, Digit Span subtest from the Wechsler Adult Intelligence Scale, Verbal Paired Associates from the Wechsler Memory Scale, and the Color Trails Test] was administered to 334 participants on enrolment and at the end of follow-up (median: 4.1 years). Multivariate analysis adjusted for confounding variables showed that the participants assigned to the Mediterranean diet + EVOO group scored higher than the controls on the RAVLT (P = 0.049) and the Color Trails Test part 2 (P = 0.04). No differences among the groups were observed for the other cognitive tests. The mean z scores of change in each test were used to construct three cognitive composites: memory, frontal (attention and executive function), and global. The adjusted changes from the baseline scores (mean z score with 95% CIs) for memory were 0.04 (-0.09 to 0.18) for the Mediterranean diet + olive oil; 0.09 (-0.05 to 0.23; P = 0.04 *vs.* controls) for the Mediterranean diet + nuts; and -0.17 (-0.32 to -0.01) for the control diet. Respective changes in frontal cognition were 0.23 (0.03 to 0.43; P = 0.003 *vs.* controls), 0.03 (-0.25 to 0.31), and -0.33 (-0.57 to -0.09). Changes in global cognition were 0.05 (-0.11 to 0.21, P = 0.005 *vs.* controls) for the Mediterranean diet + olive oil; -0.05 (-0.27 to 0.18) for the Mediterranean diet + nuts; and -0.38 (-0.57 to -0.18) for the control diet. All the cognitive composites decreased significantly (P < 0.05) on follow-up testing. The conclusion reached was that in an older population, a Mediterranean diet supplemented with olive oil or nuts was associated with improved cognitive function [53].

Outside the Mediterranean region, in Australia, a randomized controlled study (the MedLey study) assessed 137 men and women over a six-month period. Participants were randomly assigned to follow a Mediterranean diet or to maintain their customary diet. A full neuropsychological evaluation performed on enrolment and at follow-up and multivariate analysis did not disclose any significant differences between the two groups. It was therefore concluded that intervention with a Mediterranean diet had not demonstrated any beneficial effect on cognitive function in healthy older adults [54].

Finally, it may be of interest to consider the possible mechanism of the potential positive association between the Mediterranean diet and enhanced cognitive function. First, enhanced control of vascular risk factors could play an important role [55]. Second, major components in the Mediterranean diet such as fruits, vegetables, and olive oil have an antioxidant effect [24, 56]. Lastly, the diet may have an anti-inflammatory effect because of, *inter alia*, the high intake of fish and olive oil high in omega 3 fatty acids [56].

Other Dietary Patterns

The combined DASH (Dietary Approaches to Stop Hypertension) diet emphasizes the intake of fruits, vegetables, and low-fat dairy products and includes whole grains, poultry, fish, and nuts, along with reduced intake of fats, red meats, sweets, and sugary drinks [57]. The Cache County Study on Memory, Health, and Aging was a prospective population-based study that included 3,831 participants aged 65 years or above. Associations between the DASH diet and the Mediterranean diet and cognitive changes were examined. Cognitive function was evaluated using the Modified Mini-Mental State Examination (3MS) on up to four occasions over 11 years. Diet adherence index scores were calculated. Higher adherence index scores for both diets were significantly related to higher 3MS scores, and so it was concluded that greater adherence to the DASH diet and to the Mediterranean diet were associated with improved cognitive performance over 11 years [57].

Another prospective population-based study conducted in Chicago, the Memory and Aging Project (MAP), had 826 older participants and a four-year follow-up period. A neuropsychological evaluation was carried out using a battery of 19 neuropsychological tests, and the study concluded that both the DASH diet and the Mediterranean diet were significantly related to slower rates of cognitive decline in a cohort of the elderly [37].

In the Exercise and Nutrition Interventions for Cardiovascular Health (ENCORE) interventional study, 124 hypertensive, overweight subjects were randomly assigned to follow just the DASH diet, the DASH diet and a weight-loss program that included calorie restriction and physical exercise, or their habitual diet and lifestyle [58]. The neuropsychological evaluation included tests assessing executive function, memory, learning, and psychomotor speed on enrolment and at follow-up four months later. The participants in the DASH diet plus a behavioural weight control program group experienced significant enhancement in executive function-memory-learning (Cohen's D=0.562; P=0.008) and psychomotor speed (Cohen's D= 0.480; P = 0.023), while participants in the DASH diet group displayed significantly improved psychomotor speed (Cohen's D=0.440; P=0.036) compared to the control group that continued its customary diet [58].

In view of the results obtained for the Mediterranean and DASH diets, studies have been carried out seeking to ascertain which components of those diets have neuroprotective effects [59]. Researchers at Rush University therefore designed a MIND (Mediterranean-DASH Diet Intervention for Neurodegenerative Delay) diet aimed at protecting the brain, a combination of the Mediterranean and DASH diets emphasizing the intake of natural plant-based foods and limiting the intake of foods of animal origin high in saturated fats [59]. In particular, the MIND diet included foods that had exhibited some evidence of benefit to cognition, *e.g.*, leafy green vegetables, extra virgin olive oil, nuts, whole grains, legumes, and poultry. However, it did not boost fruit intake and merely recommended eating fish at least once a week [59]. A total of 960 participants in the Rush Memory and Aging Project (MAP) were followed for 4.7 years [60]. A MIND diet score that included 10 food groups that were theoretically beneficial and a further five that were theoretically detrimental to cognition was designed. The neuropsychological evaluation included tests to assess episodic memory, working memory, semantic memory, visual-spatial ability, and perceptual speed, performed at baseline and yearly. In adjusted mixed models, the MIND score was positively associated with a significantly slower decrease in the global cognitive score and in the scores for each of the five cognitive domains. The relative effects of the MIND diet and the Mediterranean and DASH diet scores on cognitive decline were compared. The MIND diet score was a better predictor of cognitive decline than either of the other diet scores; the standardized β coefficient values for the estimated effects of the diets were 4.39 for the MIND diet, 2.46 for the Mediterranean diet, and 2.60 for the DASH diet. Statistically, the correlation between the MIND diet score and cognitive change was significantly higher compared to those for the Mediterranean diet (p = 0.02) and the DASH diet (p = 0.03) [60]. The incidence of AD in that same population was also studied [61]. A total of 923 participants ranging in age from 58 to 98 years were followed for an average of 4.5 years.

Models adjusted for different variables indicated that the participants in the top tertile of MIND diet scores had a lower incidence of AD (HR: 0.47; 95% CI: 0.29 - 0.76) compared to participants in the lowest tertile. The participants in the middle tertile of MIND diet scores exhibited a statistically significant reduction in the incidence of AD compared to participants in the first tertile (HR: 0.65; 95% CI: 0.44 - 0.98). Only the top tertiles of the DASH diet and Mediterranean diet scores were significantly associated with a lower incidence of AD, as compared with the lower tertile scores. It was therefore concluded that a high degree of adherence to the MIND, DASH, and Mediterranean diets could lower the risk of AD. Moderate adherence to the MIND diet may also reduce the risk [61].

As previously mentioned, the Uppsala study in Sweden was carried out on adult men [48]. A modified MedDietS was used to evaluate adherence to the Mediterranean diet, but a modified WHO recommended diet (Healthy Diet Indicator, HDI) and a low carbohydrate high protein diet (LCHP) were also evaluated. The onset of AD, all types of dementia, and cognitive decline over 12 years were assessed, but no associations were found between any type of cognitive dysfunction and any of the dietary patterns considered.

NUTRIENTS AND THE PREVENTION OF ALZHEIMER'S DISEASE

A series of different macro and micronutrients have been examined in recent years, but to date no conclusive results backing recommendations to supplement the diet with any of these nutrients to prevent AD have been recorded [62]. The major findings in this connection are set out below.

The B-complex vitamins are involved in cell metabolism. Specifically, vitamins B6, B9 (folate), and B12 have been implicated in cognition [62]. Vitamin B9 and B12 deficiency raises blood homocysteine levels and this can lead to neurotoxicity and plaque activation and the concomitant increased risk of cerebrovascular disease [62]. Vitamin B12 deficiency has been implicated in the onset of certain cognitive and psychiatric alterations [55]. There are no conclusive data backing an association between vitamin B9 or B6 deficiency and cognitive impairment or dementia [62]. O'Leary and colleagues published a systematic literature review of studies dealing with vitamin B12, cognitive impairment, and dementia [63]. Thirty-five prospective cohort studies (14,325 subjects) were included. No evidence of any association between low serum levels of vitamin B12 and cognitive decline or dementia was found. However, four studies using vitamin B12 biomarkers [methylmalonic acid and holotranscobalamin (holoTC)] revealed an association between low vitamin B12 levels and an increased risk of cognitive impairment or dementia [63]. It should also be noted that there appears to be a relationship between elevated homocysteine levels and increased cognitive decline [62]. Meanwhile, clinical trials using vitamin B12, B6, and B9 supplementation have shown that homocysteine levels fell but that this drop was not necessarily accompanied by enhanced cognition [64].

Oxidative stress has been implicated in a range of neurodegenerative diseases, including AD, in recent years. It can result in cell damage that leads to synaptic loss and neuronal death [62]. It is therefore readily comprehensible that diverse nutrients having antioxidative properties have been regarded as holding out potentially beneficial action against neurodegeneration. These nutrients include flavonoids and vitamin C, though the findings of the studies performed have not been conclusive [62], particularly for vitamin E, the vitamin that has been studied the most. It consists of four tocopherols (α, γ, δ, and β) and their corresponding tocotrienols [55]. The prospective population-based HANDLS study included a neuropsychological evaluation and an assessment of nutritional intake at the outset. Analysis of the data for this cross-section of 1,274 subjects from 30 to 64 years of age indicated that higher vitamin E intake was associated with enhanced verbal memory, immediate memory, and verbal fluency performance, especially in younger persons [65]. However, a Cochrane systematic review turned up no conclusive results supporting vitamin E supplementation. Three studies met the inclusion criteria, two on AD patients and another on mild cognitive impairment [66].

Dietary fatty acids are ordinarily classified as saturated (mainly present in meat and dairy products) and unsaturated fatty acids (UFAs). UFAs are divided into monounsaturated (MUFAs) and polyunsaturated (PUFAs) fatty acids, chief among these being the n-3 and n-6 PUFAs (omega-3 and omega-6 fatty acids). Omega-3 fatty acids [eicosapentaenoic acid (EPA), docosahexaenoic acid (DHA), and α-linoleic acid (ALA)] are chiefly found in fish, and omega-6 fatty acids (*e.g.,* linolenic acid and arachidonic acid) are mainly present in legumes, walnuts, and other vegetable sources [67].

The human body cannot synthesize omega-3 fatty acids, making them an essential component of the diet [62]. The brain is basically made up of lipids, and DHA is the most abundant omega-3 fatty acid in the brain [62]. Saturated fatty acid intake has been associated with greater cognitive decline in prospective population-based studies [68]. Conversely, another study of 2,251 subjects with hypertension or dyslipidemia found that elevated plasma levels of n-3 PUFAs were associated with a reduction in verbal fluency decline [67].

Various observational studies have reported that a lower incidence of dementia is associated with PUFA intake [67]. Zeng and colleagues recently published a systematic literature review and concluded that higher fish consumption was significantly related to a lesser risk of AD. However, there was no statistically significant association between n-3 PUFAs, DHA, or EPA and the risk of cognitive decline [69]. Solfrizzi and colleagues reported the results of a longitudinal study carried out in Italy with three years' follow-up; they found that higher PUFA intake exhibited a protective effect against mild cognitive decline, though these findings should be viewed with caution because the number of subjects was small [70]. On the other hand, according to the results of the Rotterdam study on a cohort of 5,395 participants and follow-up for six years, high consumption of total fat, saturated fats, trans fats, or cholesterol and low consumption of MUFAs, PUFAs, n-6 PUFAs, and n-3 PUFAs was not associated with a higher risk of developing dementia [71].

None of the interventional studies published has reported positive results [67]. A Cochrane systematic review of randomized controlled studies has evaluated the efficacy of supplementation with omega-3 fatty acids in preventing cognitive decline in cognitively healthy subjects [72], and others have examined the safety and efficacy of that same supplementation in the treatment of dementia patients (including patients with AD) [73]. Each of the reviews included three randomized trials and concluded that cognitive function did not benefit from omega-3 fatty acid supplementation [72] and that there were no conclusive findings that allowed such supplementation to be recommended for treating patients with mild to moderate AD [73].

Certain clinical trials have yielded partially positive findings. Freund-Levi and colleagues published the results of a double-blind randomly controlled clinical trial and reported that administering omega-3 fatty acids (EPA and DHA) did not slow cognitive decline in patients with mild to moderate AD, though in patients with very mild AD, *i.e.*, an MMSE score > 27, cognitive decline was significantly lower in the treatment group than in the placebo group [74]. In another double-blind randomly controlled clinical trial, 50 patients over 65 years of age with mild cognitive impairment were assigned to groups treated with EPA, DHA, or n-6 linoleic acid PUFA and followed for six months. The DHA group experienced a significant improvement in verbal fluency, and the DHA and EPA groups exhibited a significant reduction in the symptoms of depression [75].

NUTRITION IN THE TREATMENT OF ALZHEIMER'S DISEASE

To date interventional studies involving supplementing the diets of AD patients with isolated nutrients have not obtained results that are sufficiently conclusive to enable any firm recommendations to be made [76]. A recent systematic review and meta-analysis of clinical trials published through 2014 evaluated the effect of supplementation with certain nutrients (antioxidants, vitamin B, inositol, medium-chain triglycerides, omega-3, polymeric formulas, a polypeptide, and vitamin D) on patients with AD in comparison with a placebo [77]. Generally speaking, studies have provided evidence for some benefits in cognition but not for Alzheimer's disease outcomes, though they have not been particularly long; nor have they had large numbers of patients, while certain studies have not used individual nutrients, like the studies on the vitamin B complex as a whole or on polymeric formulas. The conclusion reached was that supplementation with certain individual nutrients did not have a significant clinical or neuropathological effect on AD [77].

In one open clinical trial with a small number of AD patients (12) treated using acetylcholinesterase inhibitors, supplementation with vitamins C and E was provided over a year. These patients' cognitive progression was compared with that of another 11 patients in the control group treated with acetylcholinesterase inhibitors alone, without supplementation, and no significant differences were found [78]. Other clinical trials on AD patients undergoing pharmacological treatment supplemented with such nutrients as folic acid, PUFAs, and combinations of various antioxidants, generally with a small number of participants, likewise have not reported any conclusive findings [76].

One such nutrient combination is Axona®, a medium chain triglyceride product (a combination of glycerine and caprylic acid) designed to supply the brain with ketone bodies as an alternative energy source to glucose [62]. One randomized clinical trial did not find any significant differences in cognition or in any other aspect in patients with mild to moderate AD [62].

Souvenaid® is a medical food containing Fortasyn Connect, designed to enhance synapse formation in the early stages of Alzheimer's disease [62, 76]. Fortasyn Connect is a 125-ml drink that contains omega-3 PUFAs (EPA and DHA), uridine monophosphate, choline, phospholipids, and other cofactors (vitamins E, C, B12, B6, folic acid, selenium). Two clinical trials in patients with mild AD otherwise untreated, one lasting 12 weeks and the other 24 weeks, reported a significant improvement in memory [79, 80]. However, in another double-blind clinical trial over 24 weeks performed on 527 patients with mild to moderate AD undergoing pharmacological treatment, there was no evidence of cognitive improvement [81]. In an article published in 2017, Cummings and colleagues reported that the effect size of Souvenaid® was mild-moderate (Cohen's D between 0.2 and 0.5) and that its safety and tolerability profile was good, and they suggested that one out of every six Souvenaid® users will obtain a clinically detectable memory benefit [82].

CONCLUDING REMARKS

Alzheimer's disease is complex in its pathophysiology; hence lifestyle and nutrition appear to be capable of exerting a major effect on its development and progression. Numerous studies have been carried out seeking to demonstrate this. Nevertheless, despite the association between certain dietary patterns and enhanced cognitive function or even a lower incidence of dementia (including AD) found by longitudinal cohort studies, it is not possible to establish any causal relationship without interventional studies. This association may be affected by multiple factors, such as patient age or even the dementia diagnosis itself. While randomized trials on the Mediterranean diet and the DASH diet have found that greater adherence to the diet is associated with better cognitive performance, clinical trials on supplementation with individual nutrients have not repeated these same positive findings. Given that dietary patterns supply nutrients as a group, this raises the possibility that administering combinations of nutrients may yield better results and even achieve a synergistic effect. Accordingly, supplying combinations of certain nutrients that are theoretically beneficial to brain activity has been tested. This has given rise to medical foods designed to treat AD, with promising results.

As a final conclusion, the results of longitudinal cohort studies on the Mediterranean diet, the DASH diet, and the MIND diet can be said to support the view that these diets contain foods that are theoretically beneficial to brain function and that following one of these diets is important. The findings suggest that it might be possible to slow cognitive decline or even reduce the incidence of dementia and AD. Randomized trials on the Mediterranean diet and the DASH diet have likewise attested to the beneficial effects on cognitive function. Medical foods for treating mild AD have shown promising results and have exhibited a good safety and tolerability profile.

With all the above in mind, the need for clinical trials with large numbers of patients and extended duration should be underlined to enable us to properly establish the role of dietary patterns and supplementation with nutrients, individually or in combination, in the prevention and treatment of AD.

CONSENT FOR PUBLICATION

Not applicable.

CONFLICTS OF INTEREST

None declared

ACKNOWLEDGEMENTS

None declared

REFERENCES

[1]   Braak H, Braak E. Neuropathological stageing of Alzheimer-related changes. Acta Neuropathol 1991; 82(4): 239-59.
[http://dx.doi.org/10.1007/BF00308809] [PMID: 1759558]

[2]   Mirra SS, Heyman A, McKeel D, *et al.* The Consortium to Establish a Registry for Alzheimer's Disease (CERAD). Part II. Standardization of the Neuropathologic Assessment of Alzheimer's Disease. Neurology 1991; 41(4): 479-86.
[http://dx.doi.org/10.1212/WNL.41.4.479] [PMID: 2011243]

[3]   Hyman BT, Phelps CH, Beach TG, *et al.* National Institute on Aging-Alzheimer's Association guidelines for the neuropathologic assessment of Alzheimer's disease. Alzheimers Dement 2012; 8(1): 1-13.
[http://dx.doi.org/10.1016/j.jalz.2011.10.007] [PMID: 22265587]

[4]   Serrano-Pozo A, Frosch MP, Masliah E, Hyman BT. Neuropathological alterations in Alzheimer disease. Cold Spring Harb Perspect Med 2011; 1(1): a006189.
[http://dx.doi.org/10.1101/cshperspect.a006189] [PMID: 22229116]

[5]   Sperling RA, Aisen PS, Beckett LA, *et al.* Toward defining the preclinical stages of Alzheimer's disease: recommendations from the National Institute on Aging-Alzheimer's Association workgroups on diagnostic guidelines for Alzheimer's disease. Alzheimers Dement 2011; 7(3): 280-92.
[http://dx.doi.org/10.1016/j.jalz.2011.03.003] [PMID: 21514248]

[6]   American Psychiatric Association. Diagnostic and statistical manual of mental disorders (IV-TR). 4th., Washington, DC 2000.

[7]   McKhann G, Drachman D, Folstein M, Katzman R, Price D, Stadlan EM. Clinical diagnosis of Alzheimer's disease—report of the NINCDS–ADRDA work group under the auspices of Department of Health and Human Services Task Force on Alzheimer's disease. Neurology 1984; 34(7): 939-44.
[http://dx.doi.org/10.1212/WNL.34.7.939] [PMID: 6610841]

[8]   Winblad B, Palmer K, Kivipelto M, *et al.* Mild cognitive impairment--beyond controversies, towards a consensus: report of the International Working Group on Mild Cognitive Impairment. J Intern Med 2004; 256(3): 240-6.
[http://dx.doi.org/10.1111/j.1365-2796.2004.01380.x] [PMID: 15324367]

[9]   Petersen RC. Mild Cognitive impairment. Continuum (Minneap Minn) 2016; 22(2 Dementia): 404-18. [Minneap Minn].
[PMID: 27042901]

[10]   Diagnostic and statistical manual of mental disorders. 5th ed., Arlington, VA: American Psychiatric Association 2013.

[11]   McKhann GM, Knopman DS, Chertkow H, *et al.* The diagnosis of dementia due to Alzheimer's disease: recommendations from the National Institute on Aging-Alzheimer's Association workgroups on diagnostic guidelines for Alzheimer's disease. Alzheimers Dement 2011; 7(3): 263-9.
[http://dx.doi.org/10.1016/j.jalz.2011.03.005] [PMID: 21514250]

[12]   Scheltens P, Blennow K, Breteler MMB, *et al.* Alzheimer's disease. Lancet 2016; 388(10043): 505-17.
[http://dx.doi.org/10.1016/S0140-6736(15)01124-1] [PMID: 26921134]

[13]   Dubois B, Feldman HH, Jacova C, *et al.* Research criteria for the diagnosis of Alzheimer's disease: revising the NINCDS-ADRDA criteria. Lancet Neurol 2007; 6(8): 734-46.
[http://dx.doi.org/10.1016/S1474-4422(07)70178-3] [PMID: 17616482]

[14] Albert MS, DeKosky ST, Dickson D, *et al.* The diagnosis of mild cognitive impairment due to Alzheimer's disease: recommendations from the National Institute on Aging-Alzheimer's Association workgroups on diagnostic guidelines for Alzheimer's disease. Alzheimers Dement 2011; 7(3): 270-9. [http://dx.doi.org/10.1016/j.jalz.2011.03.008] [PMID: 21514249]

[15] McKhann GM, Knopman DS, Chertkow H, *et al.* The diagnosis of dementia due to Alzheimer's disease: recommendations from the National Institute on Aging-Alzheimer's Association workgroups on diagnostic guidelines for Alzheimer's disease. Alzheimers Dement 2011; 7(3): 263-9. [http://dx.doi.org/10.1016/j.jalz.2011.03.005] [PMID: 21514250]

[16] Dubois B, Feldman HH, Jacova C, *et al.* Advancing research diagnostic criteria for Alzheimer's disease: the IWG-2 criteria. Lancet Neurol 2014; 13(6): 614-29. [http://dx.doi.org/10.1016/S1474-4422(14)70090-0] [PMID: 24849862]

[17] Prince M, Wimo A, Guerchet M, Ali GC, Wu YT, Prina M. Alzheimer's Disease International. World Alzheimer Report 2015. The Global Impact of Dementia. An analysis of prevalence, incidence, cost and trends. Available from: https://www.alz.co.uk/research/WorldAlzheimer Report2015.pdf

[18] Plassman BL, Langa KM, Fisher GG, *et al.* Prevalence of cognitive impairment without dementia in the United States. Ann Intern Med 2008; 148(6): 427-34. [http://dx.doi.org/10.7326/0003-4819-148-6-200803180-00005] [PMID: 18347351]

[19] Prince M, Albanese E, Guerchet M, Prina M. Alzheimer's Disease International. World Alzheimer Report 2014. Dementia and Risk Reduction. Available from: https://www. alz. co. uk/ research/ World Alzheimer Report 2014.pdf

[20] Santos CY, Snyder PJ, Wu WC, Zhang M, Echeverria A, Alber J. Pathophysiologic relationship between Alzheimer's disease, cerebrovascular disease, and cardiovascular risk: A review and synthesis. Alzheimers Dement (Amst) 2017; 7: 69-87. [http://dx.doi.org/10.1016/j.dadm.2017.01.005] [PMID: 28275702]

[21] Solomon A, Mangialasche F, Richard E, *et al.* Advances in the prevention of Alzheimer's disease and dementia. J Intern Med 2014; 275(3): 229-50. [http://dx.doi.org/10.1111/joim.12178] [PMID: 24605807]

[22] De Bruijn RF, Bos MJ, Portegies ML, *et al.* The potential for prevention of dementia across two decades: the prospective, population-based Rotterdam Study. BMC Med 2015; 13: 132. [http://dx.doi.org/10.1186/s12916-015-0377-5] [PMID: 26195085]

[23] Gillette Guyonnet S, Abellan Van Kan G, Andrieu S, *et al.* IANA task force on nutrition and cognitive decline with aging. J Nutr Health Aging 2007; 11(2): 132-52. [PMID: 17435956]

[24] Trichopoulou A, Kouris-Blazos A, Wahlqvist ML, *et al.* Diet and overall survival in elderly people. BMJ 1995; 311(7018): 1457-60. [http://dx.doi.org/10.1136/bmj.311.7018.1457] [PMID: 8520331]

[25] Trichopoulou A, Costacou T, Bamia C, Trichopoulos D. Adherence to a Mediterranean diet and survival in a Greek population. N Engl J Med 2003; 348(26): 2599-608. [http://dx.doi.org/10.1056/NEJMoa025039] [PMID: 12826634]

[26] Panagiotakos DB, Pitsavos C, Arvaniti F, Stefanadis C. Adherence to the Mediterranean food pattern predicts the prevalence of hypertension, hypercholesterolemia, diabetes and obesity, among healthy adults; the accuracy of the MedDietScore. Prev Med 2007; 44(4): 335-40. [http://dx.doi.org/10.1016/j.ypmed.2006.12.009] [PMID: 17350085]

[27] Psaltopoulou T, Kyrozis A, Stathopoulos P, Trichopoulos D, Vassilopoulos D, Trichopoulou A. Diet, physical activity and cognitive impairment among elders: the EPIC-Greece cohort (European Prospective Investigation into Cancer and Nutrition). Public Health Nutr 2008; 11(10): 1054-62. [http://dx.doi.org/10.1017/S1368980007001607] [PMID: 18205988]

[28] Féart C, Samieri C, Rondeau V, *et al.* Adherence to a Mediterranean diet, cognitive decline, and risk

of dementia. JAMA 2009; 302(6): 638-48.
[http://dx.doi.org/10.1001/jama.2009.1146] [PMID: 19671905]

[29]   Tangney CC, Kwasny MJ, Li H, Wilson RS, Evans DA, Morris MC. Adherence to a Mediterranean-type dietary pattern and cognitive decline in a community population. Am J Clin Nutr 2011; 93(3): 601-7.
[http://dx.doi.org/10.3945/ajcn.110.007369] [PMID: 21177796]

[30]   Dietary guidelines for Americans 2005. Available from: https://health.gov/dietaryguidelines/

[31]   Kesse-Guyot E, Andreeva VA, Lassale C, *et al.* Mediterranean diet and cognitive function: a French study. Am J Clin Nutr 2013; 97(2): 369-76.
[http://dx.doi.org/10.3945/ajcn.112.047993] [PMID: 23283500]

[32]   Galbete C, Toledo E, Toledo JB, *et al.* Mediterranean diet and cognitive function: the SUN project. J Nutr Health Aging 2015; 19(3): 305-12.
[http://dx.doi.org/10.1007/s12603-015-0441-z] [PMID: 25732216]

[33]   Trichopoulou A, Kyrozis A, Rossi M, *et al.* Mediterranean diet and cognitive decline over time in an elderly Mediterranean population. Eur J Nutr 2015; 54(8): 1311-21.
[http://dx.doi.org/10.1007/s00394-014-0811-z] [PMID: 25482573]

[34]   Wengreen H, Munger RG, Cutler A, *et al.* Prospective study of dietary approaches to stop hypertension- and Mediterranean-style dietary patterns and age-related cognitive change: The cache county study on memory, health and aging. Am J Clin Nutr 2013; 98(5): 1263-71.
[http://dx.doi.org/10.3945/ajcn.112.051276] [PMID: 24047922]

[35]   Tsivgoulis G, Judd S, Letter AJ, *et al.* Adherence to a Mediterranean diet and risk of incident cognitive impairment. Neurology 2013; 80(18): 1684-92.
[http://dx.doi.org/10.1212/WNL.0b013e3182904f69] [PMID: 23628929]

[36]   Koyama A, Houston DK, Simonsick EM, *et al.* Association between the Mediterranean diet and cognitive decline in a biracial population. J Gerontol A Biol Sci Med Sci 2015; 70(3): 354-9.
[http://dx.doi.org/10.1093/gerona/glu097] [PMID: 24994847]

[37]   Tangney CC, Li H, Wang Y, *et al.* Relation of DASH- and Mediterranean-like dietary patterns to cognitive decline in older persons. Neurology 2014; 83(16): 1410-6.
[http://dx.doi.org/10.1212/WNL.0000000000000884] [PMID: 25230996]

[38]   Qin B, Adair LS, Plassman BL, *et al.* Dietary patterns and cognitive decline among Chinese older adults. Epidemiology 2015; 26(5): 758-68.
[http://dx.doi.org/10.1097/EDE.0000000000000338] [PMID: 26133024]

[39]   Cherbuin N, Anstey KJ. The Mediterranean diet is not related to cognitive change in a large prospective investigation: the PATH Through Life study. Am J Geriatr Psychiatry 2012; 20(7): 635-9.
[http://dx.doi.org/10.1097/JGP.0b013e31823032a9] [PMID: 21937919]

[40]   Gardener SL, Rainey-Smith SR, Barnes MB, *et al.* Dietary patterns and cognitive decline in an Australian study of ageing. Mol Psychiatry 2015; 20(7): 860-6.
[http://dx.doi.org/10.1038/mp.2014.79] [PMID: 25070537]

[41]   Haring B, Wu C, Mossavar-Rahmani Y, *et al.* No association between dietary patterns and risk for cognitive decline in older women with 9-year follow-up: Data from the women's health initiative memory study. J Acad Nutr Diet 2016; 116(6): 921-930.e1.
[http://dx.doi.org/10.1016/j.jand.2015.12.017] [PMID: 27050728]

[42]   Samieri C, Okereke OI, E Devore E, Grodstein F. Long-term adherence to the Mediterranean diet is associated with overall cognitive status, but not cognitive decline, in women. J Nutr 2013; 143(4): 493-9.
[http://dx.doi.org/10.3945/jn.112.169896] [PMID: 23365105]

[43]   Samieri C, Grodstein F, Rosner BA, *et al.* Mediterranean diet and cognitive function in older age. Epidemiology 2013; 24(4): 490-9.

[http://dx.doi.org/10.1097/EDE.0b013e318294a065] [PMID: 23676264]

[44] Vercambre MN, Grodstein F, Berr C, Kang JH. Mediterranean diet and cognitive decline in women with cardiovascular disease or risk factors. J Acad Nutr Diet 2012; 112(6): 816-23.
[http://dx.doi.org/10.1016/j.jand.2012.02.023] [PMID: 22709809]

[45] Scarmeas N, Stern Y, Tang MX, Mayeux R, Luchsinger JA. Mediterranean diet and risk for Alzheimer's disease. Ann Neurol 2006; 59(6): 912-21.
[http://dx.doi.org/10.1002/ana.20854] [PMID: 16622828]

[46] Scarmeas N, Stern Y, Mayeux R, Manly JJ, Schupf N, Luchsinger JA. Mediterranean diet and mild cognitive impairment. Arch Neurol 2009; 66(2): 216-25.
[http://dx.doi.org/10.1001/archneurol.2008.536] [PMID: 19204158]

[47] Gu Y, Luchsinger JA, Stern Y, Scarmeas N. Mediterranean diet, inflammatory and metabolic biomarkers, and risk of Alzheimer's disease. J Alzheimers Dis 2010; 22(2): 483-92.
[http://dx.doi.org/10.3233/JAD-2010-100897] [PMID: 20847399]

[48] Olsson E, Karlström B, Kilander L, Byberg L, Cederholm T, Sjögren P. Dietary patterns and cognitive dysfunction in a 12-year follow-up study of 70 year old men. J Alzheimers Dis 2015; 43(1): 109-19.
[http://dx.doi.org/10.3233/JAD-140867] [PMID: 25062901]

[49] Wu L, Sun D. Adherence to Mediterranean diet and risk of developing cognitive disorders: An updated systematic review and meta-analysis of prospective cohort studies. Scientific Reports 2017; 7(1): 41317.

[50] Martínez-Lapiscina EH, Clavero P, Toledo E, *et al.* Mediterranean diet improves cognition: the PREDIMED-NAVARRA randomised trial. J Neurol Neurosurg Psychiatry 2013; 84(12): 1318-25.
[http://dx.doi.org/10.1136/jnnp-2012-304792] [PMID: 23670794]

[51] Blesa R, Pujol M, Aguilar M, *et al.* Clinical validity of the 'mini-mental state' for Spanish speaking communities. Neuropsychologia 2001; 39(11): 1150-7.
[http://dx.doi.org/10.1016/S0028-3932(01)00055-0] [PMID: 11527552]

[52] Del Ser Quijano T, García de Yébenes MJ, Sánchez Sánchez F, *et al.* [Cognitive assessment in the elderly. Normative data of a Spanish population sample older than 70 years]. Med Clin (Barc) 2004; 122(19): 727-40.
[http://dx.doi.org/10.1157/13062190] [PMID: 15171906]

[53] Valls-Pedret C, Sala-Vila A, Serra-Mir M, *et al.* Mediterranean diet and age-related cognitive decline: A randomized clinical trial. JAMA Intern Med 2015; 175(7): 1094-103.
[http://dx.doi.org/10.1001/jamainternmed.2015.1668] [PMID: 25961184]

[54] Knight A, Bryan J, Wilson C, Hodgson JM, Davis CR, Murphy KJ. The Mediterranean Diet and Cognitive Function among Healthy Older Adults in a 6-Month Randomised Controlled Trial: The MedLey Study. Nutrients 2016; 8(9): E579.
[http://dx.doi.org/10.3390/nu8090579] [PMID: 27657119]

[55] Solfrizzi V, Custodero C, Lozupone M, *et al.* Relationships of Dietary Patterns, Foods, and Micro- and Macronutrients with Alzheimer's Disease and Late-Life Cognitive Disorders: A Systematic Review. J Alzheimers Dis 2017; 59(3): 815-49.
[http://dx.doi.org/10.3233/JAD-170248] [PMID: 28697569]

[56] Aridi YS, Walker JL, Wright ORL. The Association between the Mediterranean Dietary Pattern and Cognitive Health: A Systematic Review. Nutrients 2017; 9(7): E674.
[http://dx.doi.org/10.3390/nu9070674] [PMID: 28657600]

[57] Wengreen H, Munger RG, Cutler A, *et al.* Prospective study of Dietary Approaches to Stop Hypertension- and Mediterranean-style dietary patterns and age-related cognitive change: the Cache County Study on Memory, Health and Aging. Am J Clin Nutr 2013; 98(5): 1263-71.
[http://dx.doi.org/10.3945/ajcn.112.051276] [PMID: 24047922]

[58] Smith PJ, Blumenthal JA, Babyak MA, *et al.* Effects of the dietary approaches to stop hypertension

diet, exercise, and caloric restriction on neurocognition in overweight adults with high blood pressure. Hypertension 2010; 55(6): 1331-8.
[http://dx.doi.org/10.1161/HYPERTENSIONAHA.109.146795] [PMID: 20305128]

[59]   Morris MC. Nutrition and risk of dementia: overview and methodological issues. Ann N Y Acad Sci 2016; 1367(1): 31-7.
[http://dx.doi.org/10.1111/nyas.13047] [PMID: 27116239]

[60]   Morris MC, Tangney CC, Wang Y, *et al.* MIND diet slows cognitive decline with aging. Alzheimers Dement 2015; 11(9): 1015-22.
[http://dx.doi.org/10.1016/j.jalz.2015.04.011] [PMID: 26086182]

[61]   Morris MC, Tangney CC, Wang Y, Sacks FM, Bennett DA, Aggarwal NT. MIND diet associated with reduced incidence of Alzheimer's disease. Alzheimers Dement 2015; 11(9): 1007-14.
[http://dx.doi.org/10.1016/j.jalz.2014.11.009] [PMID: 25681666]

[62]   Prince M, Albanese E, Guerchet M, Prina M. Alzheimer's Disease International. Nutrition and dementia Available from: https://wwwalzcouk/sites/default/files/pdfs/nutrition-and-dementiapdf

[63]   O'Leary F, Allman-Farinelli M, Samman S. Vitamin B_{12} status, cognitive decline and dementia: a systematic review of prospective cohort studies. Br J Nutr 2012; 108(11): 1948-61.
[http://dx.doi.org/10.1017/S0007114512004175] [PMID: 23084026]

[64]   Ford AH, Almeida OP. Effect of homocysteine lowering treatment on cognitive function: a systematic review and meta-analysis of randomized controlled trials. J Alzheimers Dis 2012; 29(1): 133-49.
[http://dx.doi.org/10.3233/JAD-2012-111739] [PMID: 22232016]

[65]   Beydoun MA, Fanelli-Kuczmarski MT, Kitner-Triolo MH, *et al.* Dietary antioxidant intake and its association with cognitive function in an ethnically diverse sample of US adults. Psychosom Med 2015; 77(1): 68-82.
[http://dx.doi.org/10.1097/PSY.0000000000000129] [PMID: 25478706]

[66]   Farina N, Isaac MG, Clark AR, Rusted J, Tabet N. Vitamin E for Alzheimer's dementia and mild cognitive impairment. Cochrane Database Syst Rev 2012; 11: CD002854.
[PMID: 23152215]

[67]   Smith PJ, Blumenthal JA. Dietary Factors and Cognitive Decline. J Prev Alzheimers Dis 2016; 3(1): 53-64.
[PMID: 26900574]

[68]   Morris MC, Evans DA, Bienias JL, Tangney CC, Wilson RS. Dietary fat intake and 6-year cognitive change in an older biracial community population. Neurology 2004; 62(9): 1573-9.
[http://dx.doi.org/10.1212/01.WNL.0000123250.82849.B6] [PMID: 15136684]

[69]   Zeng LF, Cao Y, Liang WX, *et al.* An exploration of the role of a fish-oriented diet in cognitive decline: a systematic review of the literature. Oncotarget 2017; 8(24): 39877-95.
[http://dx.doi.org/10.18632/oncotarget.16347] [PMID: 28418899]

[70]   Solfrizzi V, Colacicco AM, D'Introno A, *et al.* Dietary intake of unsaturated fatty acids and age-related cognitive decline: a 8.5-year follow-up of the Italian Longitudinal Study on Aging. Neurobiol Aging 2006; 27(11): 1694-704.
[http://dx.doi.org/10.1016/j.neurobiolaging.2005.09.026] [PMID: 16256248]

[71]   Engelhart MJ, Geerlings MI, Ruitenberg A, *et al.* Diet and risk of dementia: Does fat matter?: The Rotterdam Study. Neurology 2002; 59(12): 1915-21.
[http://dx.doi.org/10.1212/01.WNL.0000038345.77753.46] [PMID: 12499483]

[72]   Sydenham E, Dangour AD, Lim WS. Omega 3 fatty acid for the prevention of cognitive decline and dementia. Cochrane Database Syst Rev 2012; 6(6): CD005379.
[PMID: 22696350]

[73]   Burckhardt M, Herke M, Wustmann T, Watzke S, Langer G, Fink A. Omega-3 fatty acids for the treatment of dementia. Cochrane Database Syst Rev 2016; 4: CD009002.

[PMID: 27063583]

[74] Freund-Levi Y, Eriksdotter-Jönhagen M, Cederholm T, *et al.* Omega-3 fatty acid treatment in 174 patients with mild to moderate Alzheimer disease: OmegAD study: a randomized double-blind trial. Arch Neurol 2006; 63(10): 1402-8.
[http://dx.doi.org/10.1001/archneur.63.10.1402] [PMID: 17030655]

[75] Sinn N, Milte CM, Street SJ, *et al.* Effects of n-3 fatty acids, EPA v. DHA, on depressive symptoms, quality of life, memory and executive function in older adults with mild cognitive impairment: a 6-month randomised controlled trial. Br J Nutr 2012; 107(11): 1682-93.
[http://dx.doi.org/10.1017/S0007114511004788] [PMID: 21929835]

[76] Giulietti A, Vignini A, Nanetti L, Mazzanti L, Di Primio R, Salvolini E. Alzheimer's Disease Risk and Progression: The Role of Nutritional Supplements and their Effect on Drug Therapy Outcome. Curr Neuropharmacol 2016; 14(2): 177-90.
[http://dx.doi.org/10.2174/1570159X13666150928155321] [PMID: 26415975]

[77] Muñoz Fernández SS, Ivanauskas T, Lima Ribeiro SM. Nutritional Strategies in the Management of Alzheimer Disease: Systematic Review With Network Meta-Analysis. J Am Med Dir Assoc 2017; 18(10): 897.e13-30.
[http://dx.doi.org/10.1016/j.jamda.2017.06.015] [PMID: 28807434]

[78] Arlt S, Müller-Thomsen T, Beisiegel U, Kontush A. Effect of one-year vitamin C- and E-supplementation on cerebrospinal fluid oxidation parameters and clinical course in Alzheimer's disease. Neurochem Res 2012; 37(12): 2706-14.
[http://dx.doi.org/10.1007/s11064-012-0860-8] [PMID: 22878647]

[79] Scheltens P, Kamphuis PJ, Verhey FR, *et al.* Efficacy of a medical food in mild Alzheimer's disease: A randomized, controlled trial. Alzheimers Dement 2010; 6(1): 1-10.e1.
[http://dx.doi.org/10.1016/j.jalz.2009.10.003] [PMID: 20129316]

[80] Scheltens P, Twisk JWR, Blesa R, *et al.* Efficacy of Souvenaid in mild Alzheimer's disease: results from a randomized, controlled trial. J Alzheimers Dis 2012; 31(1): 225-36.
[http://dx.doi.org/10.3233/JAD-2012-121189] [PMID: 22766770]

[81] Shah RC, Kamphuis PJ, Leurgans S, *et al.* The S-Connect study: results from a randomized, controlled trial of Souvenaid in mild-to-moderate Alzheimer's disease. Alzheimers Res Ther 2013; 5(6): 59.
[http://dx.doi.org/10.1186/alzrt224] [PMID: 24280255]

[82] Cummings J, Scheltens P, McKeith I, *et al.* Effect Size Analyses of Souvenaid in Patients with Alzheimer's Disease. J Alzheimers Dis 2017; 55(3): 1131-9.
[http://dx.doi.org/10.3233/JAD-160745] [PMID: 27767993]

CHAPTER 9

Treatment and Control of Behavioral and Psychololgical Symptoms

Juan Carlos Durán Alonso[*]

Geriatric Medicine Department, "San Juan Grande" Hospital, Jerez de la Frontera, Cádiz, Spain

Abstract: The behavioral and psychological symptoms of dementia are very frequent, appearing during the evolution of the different types of dementia, generating stress for both the patient and their caregivers. They include a wide group of symptoms: agitation, irritability, aggression, hallucinations, delusions, depression, anxiety or insomnia, and need to make an individual assessment of each patient. The management of these situations requires non-pharmacological measures such as education of caregivers, physical and sensory stimulation or music therapy.

When these measures are not effective and the situation is stressful we must resort to pharmacological treatment. Different medications may be useful, but the most frequently used are antipsychotics. Having to start with low doses and evaluate efficacy and safety, and maintaining the necessary time to control the symptoms, and then schedule their progressive withdrawal.

Keywords: BPSD, Behavioral and psychological symptoms of dementia, Dementia.

INTRODUCTION

Dementia is an acquired syndrome, that could be caused by different diseases, in which memory and other intellectual functions are affected, without altering conscience level, progressive course, and which affects the ability of the individual to perform his life activities.

Many diseases can trigger dementia, with Alzheimer being the most frequent, followed by vascular dementia, and other degenerative diseases such as dementia of Lewy bodies or dementia associated with Parkinson´s disease. Dementia may appear in the course of endocrine diseases such as hypothyroidism, and deficient vitamin B12 or folic acid.

---

[*] **Corresponding author Juan Carlos Durán Alonso:** Geriatric Medicine Department, "San Juan Grande" Hospital, Jerez de la Frontera, Cádiz, Spain; Tel: +34 607694639; E-mail: juancarlos.duran@sjd.es; juancaduran@ono.com

Blas Gil-Extremera (Ed.)

While more important symptoms to the diagnostic of dementia is in the cognitive sphere, as reflected in the diagnostic criteria, this patient presents in their disease course, different psychiatric clinical manifestations, which, following the consensus conference of the International Association of Psychogeriatric in 1996, are defined as Behavioral and Psychological Symptoms of Dementia [BPSD] [1].

Refer to this group of symptoms, both the psychological symptoms: depression, anxiety, apathy, insomnia, which are symptoms developed by the patient and require a clinical assessment with both the patient and the caregiver; as well as behavioral symptoms: irritability, aggressiveness, erratic deambulation, motor hyperactivity, illusions, hallucinations and delusional ideas. Many of these symptoms are detected with patient observation [2] (Table **1**).

Table 1. Types of Behavioral and Psychological Symptoms of Dementia

BEHAVIORAL.
- Agitation:
o Repeating questions
o Inapropiate screaming, crying, disruptive sound
o Easily upset
o Leaving home
- Irritability
- Motor disturbance: wandering or rummaging
- Agression: physical or verbal
- Desinhibition: socialy or sexualy inappropriate behavioral
PSYCHOLOGICAL.
- Psychosis:
o Hallucinations
o Delusions
- Depression
- Anxiety
- Apathy or indifference
- Insomnia

The prevalence of behavioral and psychological symptoms in dementias is very high. Almost all patients [97%] have at least one of these symptoms throughout the disease. It is very frequent also that several of these symptoms, such as depression with anxiety and insomnia, or hallucinations with delusions, irritability, anxiety and aggressiveness appear in the same patient [2].

Such symptoms may appear more frequently depending on the type of dementia. Thus, in vascular dementias, depression is more frequent; in Lewy bodies the hallucinations, and apathy and disinhibiting in the frontotemporal dementia [2].

The behavioural and psychological symptoms may occur during any phase of dementia, but depression and anxiety are more common in the early stages, while psychosis, agitation, and aggressiveness appear in later stages [3].

On the other hand there are symptoms that are more enduring in time, like apathy, while others occur in a very punctual or very acute way like the hallucinations, aggressiveness or catastrophic reactions [3].

Behavioral and psychological symptoms produce great suffering in the patient, deteriorating their quality of life and generating a marked stress and burnout in their carregivers. In fact, many studies have shown that the higher socio-sanitary cost generated by dementias are due to these behavioral and psychological symptoms, since they motivate numerous medical consultations, and generate a need for resources: need to hire professional caregivers at home, go to day units or institutionalization of the patient in geriatric center [1 - 4].

Many papers about stress in dementias disease, describe symptoms in the caregivers, like anxiety, depression or sleep disturbances, thus reducing the quality of life and deteriorating the health status of family and caregivers of patients with dementia [1 - 4].

DIAGNOSTIC OF BEHAVIORAL AND PSYCHOLOGICAL SYMPTOMS

As it is a wide range of different symptoms, ranging from apathy to hyperactivity, or from sadness to aggressiveness, management will be different in each case, making it difficult to record, and should always be approached in an individualized way [2, 4].

We must go deeper to know the type of behavioral and psychological symptoms are prevalent in the patient, to know if it presents a concrete set of symptoms that could correlate with each other. Are to know if there is any factor or circumstance that could act as a trigger for the appearance of these symptoms [4].

To do this, we must make a complete clinical history, maintaining a structured interview with the patient and his main caregiver, to know what type of symptomatology presents, the underlying pathology of the patient and if there could be any factor that acts as a trigger process. Direct observation of the patient is important to see their attitude and behavior: uninhibited, with motor hyperactivity, or with verbal or physical aggressiveness [2 - 4].

There are different scales that can be useful to evaluate the BPSD, to see both the frequency of occurrence, the severity of the symptoms and the repercussions they have on the patient and the family. Of all the existent scales that emphasizes its universality is the NPI [Neuro Psychiatric Inventory]. It measures was published by Cummings, and evaluates in 10 items: delusions, hallucinations, agitation, depression, anxiety, euphoria, apathy, disinhibition, irritability and motor behavior without purpose, both its frequency [0 = absent, 4 = very frequent], as its severity [1 = slight: it causes little discomfort, a 3 = severe: very annoying for the patient and difficult to approach] [5]. It was later validated in Spanish by Vilalta [6].

Different authors like Lyketsos, propose to obtain an adequate classification of the BPSD in syndromes, and to select later, its treatment as well. Thus these scales, differentiate patients with predominantly affective syndrome, either depressive, agitated-anxious; and psychotic predominance syndrome [7].

Other authors, such as Petrovic, publish observational studies in six European geriatric centers, recruiting 194 patients with dementia, of whom 96% had BPSD. The most frequent were apathy (59.6%), depression (58.8%), irritability (44.6%), anxiety (44%) and agitation [41.5%], and proposed to classify BPSDs in four subgroups:

- Psychotic predominance, which includes irritability, agitation, hallucinations and anxiety

- Psychomotor Predominance: including erratic ambulation and delusions

- Predominance mood disorders: with depression, euphoria or disinhibition, and

- Instinctive predominance: with apathy, sleep disorders, and appetite disorders [8].

In many patients these symptoms may be correlated, and while the predominant symptoms may initially appear, but may trigger other types of symptoms. So patients with dementia, can initially present with depressive symptoms, and mood alterations. These can develop in to thinking disorders with delusional ideas that trigger an outbreak of agitation with verbal or physical aggressiveness (Fig. **1**).

A complex problem such as the management of the behavioral and psychological symptoms of dementia, which requires the combination of non-pharmacological treatments, together with medication with possible significant adverse effects, requires the collaboration of the entire professionals' team responsible for the care of the patient. The multidisciplinary teamwork is fundamental, with the participation not only of the doctor, also of nursing, psychology, physiotherapy and occupational therapy. Putting in common their different points of view of the patient, to create an individualized plan of care, specific for each subject with dementia and different at each moment. The plan needs to be reviewed to know the patient's response to the established treatment plan, and to be able to make modification as required.

Clustering of BPSD

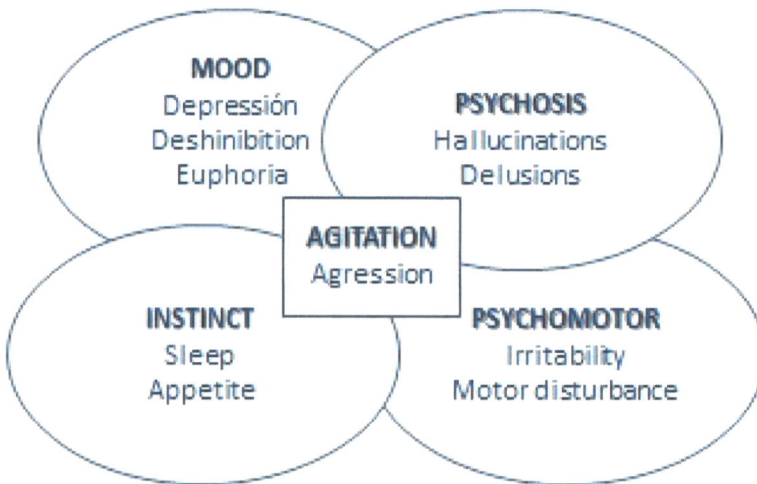

Fig. (1). BPSD: diferent symptoms.

TREATMENT OF THE CONDUCTUAL AND PSYCHOLOGICAL SYMPTOMS OF THE DEMENTIA

Non-Pharmacological Treatment

Before treating, it is essential to know each patient, since the behavioral and psychological symptoms are different according to the type of dementia, and according to the different phases of dementia in which the patient is.

First, it is important to ensure that the patient has his or her basic needs covered. The patient should not be thirsty, hungry, cold, hot, unsafe, on alone. The possibility should be considered, such us other undercurrent medical illness that could cause the symptoms: constipation or faecal impaction, urinary retention, dyspnoea or chest pain, dyspepsia, osteoarticular pain that appears with the mobilization or before a determined posture, or some infectious disease [3, 4].

It is fundamental to schedule a routine for each patient, with a specific time to get up, clean, regular meal times, napping should be less than 30 minutes, and sleeping at the same time each night.

It is also recommended a routine environment, that is familiar and comfortable, where there are spaces to move, a place to carry out activities, and a suitable place for meals, as well as a bedroom with dim lights preferably in the bathroom in case the patient wakes up at night. Patients with dementia are more compromised when they frequently change their domicile, which is a common trigger for the appearance of behavioral and psychological symptoms.

Patients with dementia suffer from an acute illness that requires hospitalization. In addition to the problems that the acute illness generates are a change in daily routine along with hospitalizaton which entails, blood extraction, dropper, or bladder catheterization, and other techniques that can cause pain and discomfort. This leads to an alteration in sleep-wake rhythm, disorientation and increased confusion. Coming in to nursing homes requires an adaptation period. Everything is new for the patient, who does not know the professional, staff the caregivers who must take care of his or her daily activities and who unknown to the patient, so can be perceived as discordant agents, which generates irritability, suspicions, and abnormal behaviors. Once institutionalized, the changes should be minimized so that the patient can move in a safe and familiar environment.

Caregivers Training

There are different modes of action, some aimed at training caregivers, both family members and professionals in nursing homes, so that they are well prepared in the management of behavioral disorders.

It is essential to know well that the different behavioral and psychological symptoms are clinical manifestations that appear as a consequence of dementia. The patient suffers from presenting these symptoms, and the primary caregiver must have sufficient skills to avoid conflict with the patient, try to divert his or her attention, keep calm and convey peace and tranquillity. As advice is transmitted to caregivers who should not raise the tone of voice, maintain eye contact with patients, and avoid position of superiority. Caregivers should not argue, and avoid uncomfortable discussions with the patient.

We must teach the patient's primary caregivers, to recognize the times of day, and concrete circumstances that can trigger the onset of psychological symptoms. The most frequent moments are those during the care of the basic activities of daily life, like using the toilet, bathing and dressing. By not recognizing of patients with dementia can be help. Patients try to keep their intimacy, and it cost them another person to help them in toilet, see them naked. As such, caregivers have can to be extremely meticulous in this moments, and have to gradually gain their confidence. Patients with dementia who suffer from incontinence require the use of absorbent diapers, and changing them also tends to be psychologically uncomfortable.

Another difficult time is during feeding. It is recommended that patients eat with the rest of the family if they live at home, or all together in the dining room if they are in a nursing home. Cognitive impairment causes them to forget when they have eaten, so they may want to eat more. Apraxia secondary to dementia leads makes it difficult for them to properly use cutlery, sometimes they eat with their hands, and can be messy, these circumstances must be accepted [1, 4, 9].

The dementia patient´s caregiver plays an essential role in the prevention of things that trigger BPSD, and can sometimes reinforce the patient's symptoms, with an excessively paternalistic, authoritarian or infantilizing treatment that can irritate the patient. The imposed orders do not usually work with the patients, nor does the repeated repetition of the demands to remind them [1, 4, 9].

Programming of Activities

There is enough scientific evidence to support that patients with dementia who suffer from behavioral and psychological symptoms improve when they spend their time engaging in physical and mental activities [1, 3 - 5, 10, 11].

Numerous scientific publications in recent years demonstrate the progressive interest in non-pharmacological treatment of behavioral disorders in patients with dementia.

Significant revisions have been made in the use of non-pharmacological interventions at both community and nursing home levels. A recent systematic overview of all reviews published in The Senator on Top series has recently been published in BMJ [11].

The programs aimed at acting directly on the patient with dementia focus on different areas: physical exercise practice, psychostimulation and psycho-relaxation programs, sensory stimulation, and musical therapies [10, 11].

In our geriatric setting we have scheduled daily activities for patients with dementias, separating the group of mild-stage dementias from another group of moderate / severe dementias. These are delivered by experts in psychology, physiotherapy and occupational therapy, collaborating in social, cultural and caregiving context.

In both groups, the day begins with a program of temporary orientation. The calendar is updated, having to orient all the patients, as day to the week, day to the month, the month and the year, as well as the season of the year. For this activity we use large posters, which are displayed in their rooms until the next day, in full view of all of them.

In the group of mild cognitive impairment and dementia in the mild phase, a daily reading session is held in the press, where a technician reads and comments with them the most outstanding news that appears in the press, trying to involve all of them in it, encovering them to comment and repeating several times, what the most outstanding or impressive parts were.

Later, we separated the groups, one of them going to the gym, where the physiotherapy team, carried out group programs of elderly-gym, for periods between 40 and 60 minutes. Here perform different activities that motivate the motor, working from the neck, shoulders, arms, back, abdomen to the lower limbs. Some patients require separate individualized treatments.

Occupational therapists perform exercises to stimulate fine psychomotricity, enhancing manual activities with a greater or lesser degree of complexity, depending on the stage of illness of each patient.

While the psychologist performs daily cognitive psycho-stimulation programs, where she alternates the stimulation of the different cognitive areas, from reading aloud workshops that we call "on the phone", expressive theatrical activities, workshops of mathematical skills, semantic workshops, where they participate with word games, crossword puzzles, soups of letters, and thematic workshops where subjects of geography, animals, plants or simple everyday objects are used to stimulate them to remember. A very specific workshop that we consider one of the most fun is the one of laughter-therapy, where everyone is encouraged to tell a joke, joke or fun event that would have had, generating shared laughter in the group and encouraging them to see who laughs more or better.

Another very effective workshop for the control of the behavioral and psychological symptoms of dementia, developed by the psychologist is the psycho-relaxation. For those who are looking for a quiet environment, with dim light and relaxing background music, teaching everyone to remain in silence for a while, playing with their breathing and muscle relaxation, making them think of places or moments that are very relaxing, sometimes many begin to fall asleep in the workshop.

Also being very useful are the workshops with music therapy and dance-therapy. We do two types of workshops, some individualized, and others in group. For the individualized we have MP3s with headphones, so that the music can be different for each patient. Previously we have investigated the musical tastes of the patient, which is very important to know, and can be obtain through his relatives, which type of music stimulates the patient most, as well as to know his or her musical biography, and the music which he or she enjoyed most in his or her youth.

Periods between 30 and 60 minutes of music therapy help reduce the most positive behavioral symptoms. Many older people sing their songs as they listen, relax, smile and become stimulated. When they are more irritable we try to put on relaxing classical music, being an occasionally effective measure for their control. The group workshops are held together in the room listening to certain melodies, and sometimes they are invited to participate with some simple musical instrument, and in others to dance.

It is in the section of music therapy where more work is being done today. Its scientific basis is that patients with dementia lose their ability to express themselves, but reminiscences remain, preserving the ability to recall musical memories to advanced stages of the disease. It can be based on the musical they are hearing or also on the musical participation trough playing some kind of instrument. Sometimes dance therapy is added to practice movements and exercises to the dance. The management must be individualized, investigating the musical tastes of the patient. The sessions must have a concrete duration. The results of the different studies have shown that they reduce both the frequency and intensity of behavioral disorders, reducing the need to use antipsychotics and anxiolytics [12, 13].

To assess the efficacy of occupational therapy to reduce symptoms of cognitive impairment and Alzheimer's disease, a study was conducted by the Occupational Therapy Working Group of the Spanish Geriatrics and Gerontology Society, where they reviewed randomized clinical trials, cohort studies, observational studies and experimental, clinical practice guidelines and systematic reviews, published between 2010 and 2015, using as bibliographic searches the main scientific databases. From the total of 139 articles, 25 were selected, concluding that non-pharmacological interventions are effective for delaying the onset of dysfunction in patients with dementia, focusing on benefits, in addition to performing their basic activities of daily living, for emotional functioning [10].

In the nursing homes, a systematic review published by Cabrera and colleagues of the Pompeu Fabra University of Barcelona, included a total of 31 publications, including randomized studies, meta-analysis and clinical guidelines, where the fundamental parameters to be analysed were quality of care or the quality of life in patients with institutionalized dementia. They concluded that although the work focused on staff training, those aimed at demented patients, included physical activity, sensory therapy and cognitive stimulation. However, the conclusion was that there is still insufficient evidence to claim that non-pharmacological measures are effective for the control of behavioral symptoms and psychological factors associated with dementia [14].

A recent publication by Hsu, studying a group of 141 elderly people with dementia in two residences in Taiwan, evaluated the predictive factors for the response to a non-pharmacological intervention with its effects on cognition and the behavioral and psychological symptoms associated with dementia. The interventions they performed with them were programs of physical exercise, orientation to reality, music therapy, reminiscences and horticulture for 6 months. They found that those who benefited most from non-pharmacological treatment were subjects with lower cognitive levels, more severe BPSD, and depressive symptoms. While the ones with the least benefit were those who were being treated with antipsychotics [15].

Pharmacological Treatment

It is a challenge for medical professionals to control BPSD in patients with dementia, thus improving their quality of life that patients and their caregivers. The control of these symptoms is complex and involves the combination of non-pharmacological measures, and in many cases accompanied by the use of psychoactive drugs.

As a first intervention, all non-pharmacological measures mentioned should be applied, reserving medications for most acute, stressful and potentially dangerous symptoms for the patient [16].

Before starting a pharmacological treatment, one must always evaluate the possible triggers that may have caused these symptoms, such as the presence of an intercurrent medical illness, including infection, chronic osteoarticular pain, dyspnea, chest tightness, constipation, fecal impaction, or urinary retention . The introduction of a new drugs that cause this symptomatology, or some new social circumstance causing, it should also be considered [3, 4, 22]. Table **2**.

Table 2. Recommendations for the Use if Antipsychotic in Patients with Dementia.

1.- Before prescribing medication, evaluate factors that can act as triggers and treat or avoid them:
- medicals [infections, pain, constipation ...]

(Table 2) cont.....

- environmental
2.- First apply non-pharmacological interventions:
- Education of caregivers.
- Psychomotricity
- Psychostimulation / Psychorelaxation
- Sensory stimulation
- Music Therapy
3. If it is a degenerative dementia type of Alzheimer's, evaluate benefit in the control of the BPSD of anticholinesterases drugs [Donepezil, rivastigmine or galantamine] or memantine.
4. To assess the initiation of treatment with haloperidol, starting at low doses and progressively adjusting, evaluating benefit in terms of symptom control, and monitoring possible occurrence of adverse effects. Schedule withdrawal when controlling them.
5. If symptoms are not controlled, haloperidol is not favourable, is not tolerated, side effects and a negative benefit-risk profiles, initiate treatment with risperidone as the only atypical antipsychotic authorized for a period of time up to 6 weeks. Initiate with low doses [0.5-1 mg / d] and increase progressively. Avoid in patients with previous cerebrovascular accidents.
6. In the case of dementia of Lewy bodies or Parkinson's dementia, quetiapine may be the drug of choice. Inform family and caregivers.

We must ensure that patients with dementia who are candidates for the use of anticholinesterase drugs or with memantine are taking them, since these drugs, in addition to stabilizing the disease in their cognitive sphere, have been shown to reduce the intensity and frequency of behavioral disorders. Specifically, the study published by Walderman, showed that donepezil reduced the occurrence of apathy, hallucinations, and improved motor hyperactivity [17]. Figiel published a systematic review to evaluate the efficacy of rivastigmine in the control of BPSD in the different types of dementia: Alzheimer's, vascular, frontotemporal, Lewy bodies and associated with Parkinson's. The symptoms that achieved significant improvement were apathy, anxiety, delusions and hallucinations [18].

Tangwongchai published a study with galantamine, whose objective was to evaluate the efficacy of this in the control of BPSD, carrying out a 6-month multicenter study, including 75 patients with Alzheimer's dementia, vascular dementia and BPSD, aiming at statistically significant improvement, especially in the improvement of delusions, anxiety, phobias and disturbances of the wake-sleep rhythm of the group treated with galantamine [19]. Grossberg demonstrated in a memantine study that it reduces the occurrence of agitation and aggressiveness in patients with moderate-severe dementia [20].

There are several pharmacological groups that we can use for psychological problems, with antipsychotics being the most frequently used. Other possible remedies are antidepressants, anxiolytics, mood stabilizers, and hypnotics.

Depending on the prevalence of BPSD type, therapeutic management will be different, requiring an individualized approach to the patient. So if mood disorders predominate, with depression or apathy, we could select an antidepressant. If anxiety predominates, an anxiolytic, an antidepressant with a sedative effect or an anticonvulsant as a mood stabilizer; and if psychotic symptoms predominate, we will select an antipsychotic to control them. Many times we have to combine drugs to achieve goals, associating antipsychotics with antidepressants, with anxiolytics or with hypnotics, which increases the risk of adverse effects, demanding greater patient vigilance (Fig. **2**).

Treatment of BPSD

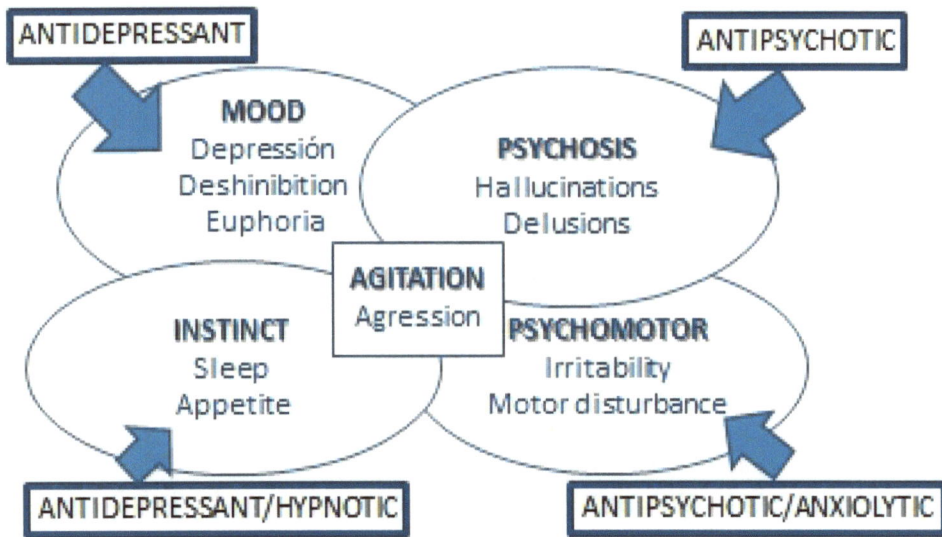

Fig. (2). BPSD: Different pharmacological treatments.

Antipsychotic Drugs

A scientific discussion on the use of antipsychotics has been created in the last decade, which has focused more on its safety than its effectiveness. Publications appeared that related the use of atypical antipsychotics with an increased risk of stroke. Subsequently other studies found that patients treated with antipsychotics had a higher mortality than those who did not. There also appeared publications indicating an increased risk of urinary or respiratory infections in patients with dementia who were taking antipsychotics, and now, it has also been published that there exist an association with an increased risk of fractures.

For these reasons, the State Regulatory Agencies on the use of medicines, both in Spain and in other countries, warned of the risk of increased stroke and death in patients with dementia treated with these drugs, especially those suffering from vascular dementia, stroke or associated vascular risk factors. The Spanish Ministry of Health included the need for a visa for the prescription of these drugs. Only patients with dementia are allowed to use haloperidol without a visa, and for risperidone with a visa, authorizing a short-term treatment of up to 6 weeks in patients with moderate to severe Alzheimer's dementia who do not respond to other non-pharmacological measures and when there is a risk of harm to them or to others without such medication [21].

All this has made the physicians that we face in our usual clinical practice who are challenged with treating these patients become more cautious in their selection of the drug. It is selected one drug that presents a better profile, more specific for each patient. They need to start with the lowest dose possible, following a stepwise progressive guideline until achieving its efficacy by adjusting doses every 5-7 days, always watching for the possible occurrence of adverse effects with the scheduling of periodic reviews. If there is no response to the drug after 2-3 weeks, we must consider another therapeutic alternative, and if the drug is effective and controls the symptoms, we should keep the treatment for as short time as possible once we reach the control of the symptoms [22, 23].

Haloperidol, a first-generation antipsychotic, has demonstrated efficacy in the treatment of aggression, and to a lesser extent in agitation. The cost of the drug is lower than atypical drug. It has extrapyramidal adverse effects and produces sedation. Longer-term use is therefore not recommended, as recommended by Lonergan's findings in a systematic review of five randomized clinical trials evaluating drug efficacy and safety published in Cochrane [24]. A 1.5-fold higher mortality risk for haloperidol compared to atypical antipsychotic drugs during the first four weeks of treatment was observed in a study published by Kales [25].

Atypical antipsychotic drugs have shown to be efficacious in different studies for control in behavioral and psychological symptoms associated with dementia. In a Cochrane review published in 2004, the efficacy and safety of atypicals were evaluated, selecting 16 studies with a minimum duration of 6 weeks, randomized, double-blind trials. The highest percentage of studies were performed with risperidone, followed by olanzapine, quetiapine and aripiprazole. They included mostly Alzheimer's patients, but some included vascular dementias or mixed dementias, with mean age between 79 and 83 years. The results showed that treatment with risperidone at doses between 1 and 2 mg / day was associated with a significant improvement symptoms and agitation with aggressiveness [26].

Subsequently, Schneider published a meta-analysis, evaluating the different, randomized, placebo-controlled, multicenter trials of atypical antipsychotics to assess their efficacy and safety. They selected 16 studies, with a total of 3,353 patients. They were 5 with risperidone, 5 with olanzapine, 3 with aripiprazole and 3 with quetiapine. They concluded that risperidone and aripiprazole showed greater efficiency, and olanzapine and risperidone had higher adverse effects, most notably drowsiness, urinary incontinence, urinary tract infections and extrapyramidal symptoms [27].

The CATIE-AD [Clinical Antipsychotic Trials of Intervention Effectiveness-Alzheimer's Disease] study, in which 42 centers, involving 421 patients with Alzheimer's disease, psychoses, aggression or agitation. Four different groups were randomized, with risperidone, olanzapine, quetiapine and placebo respectively. Doses were adjusted according to patients' needs, and follow-up was 36 weeks. They evaluated the percentage of patients who had improved: 32% with olanzapine, 29% with risperidone, 26% with quetiapine. And the mean time of suspension for loss of efficacy, being better for risperidone: 26.7 weeks, olanzapine 22.1 weeks and quetiapine 9.1 weeks. The percentage of patients who had to discontinue the study due to adverse effects was 24% olanzapine, 18% risperidone, and 16% quetiapine. They conclude that the low efficacy of atypical antipsychotics is not compensated for its habitual use with high percentages of adverse effects, and each case should be individualized [28].

We published a study: evaluation of risperidone in the treatment of behavioral and psychological symptoms and sleep disturbances in patients with dementia; being a multicenter, observational and prospective study of 12 weeks' duration, including a total of 338 patients, of which 321 completed the study. The mean dose of risperidone was 1.49 mg / d, and we used the Neuropsychiatric Inventory [NPI] and a specific scale to evaluate duration and quality of sleep, early awakenings and daytime sleepiness. We concluded that risperidone was effective for the control of the symptoms, with decrease of the NPI in 10.6 points, as well as improvement in the sleep of the patients, being well tolerated [29].

Special consideration is given to patients with Lewy body dementia, who are hypersensitive to treatment with antipsychotic drugs, worsening extrapyramidal symptoms. For this dementia group, as with the psychotic symptoms of patients with dementia associated with Parkinson's disease, the most recommended antipsychotic is quetiapine, because its better tolerance and less association with extrapyramidal effects [30]. In studies to evaluate the efficacy of rivastigmine in this subgroup of dementias, improvements in psychotic symptoms were observed, especially in hallucinations [31].

Other Drugs

Benzodiazepines are a therapeutic option for the control of anxiety, although their prolonged use in time can be associated to adverse effects, both cognitive and functional, to produce apraxia of gait, increasing the risk of falls. A rebound effect may appear, with worsening anxiety following prescription. And a dose ceiling effect has been described in elderly patients, in which, when much their dose is increased, the desired effect does not improve, however, there is worsening of adverse effects. Of the different benzodiazepines, lorazepam at doses between 0.5 and 3 mg daily is most appropriate for elderly patients with dementia, due to their intermediate half-life and hepatocyte metabolism.

When depressive symptoms predominate in the patient, it would be preferable to start treatment with antidepressants. Tricyclics should be avoided because of their anticholinergic effects that worsen cognitive functions. Selective serotonin reuptake inhibitors are the first choice. Citalopram, at doses between 10 and 20 mg has demonstrated efficacy, has few interactions, and is useful in depression associated with vasculocerebral diseases. The CITAD study [Citalopram for Agitation in Alzheimer´s disease] included 186 randomized people with clinically significant agitation who received citalopram or placebo for nine weeks. The group taking citalopram showed significant improvement on several clinical measures [32].

Trazodone is an antidepressant with an intense sedative profile, and may be useful if depression is associated with anxiety and insomnia [33]. Mirtazapine also has a sedative and hypnotic effect, and by increasing appetite and producing weight gain, it may be indicated when it is associated with insomnia and altered eating behavior with loss of appetite, a problem that often generates stress for caregivers [22].

Another pharmacological group that we can sometimes resort to when neuroleptic treatment fails, are antiepileptics, used in psychiatry as mood stabilizers, and clinical trials performed to control symptoms in dementias. Of these, carbamazepine demonstrated efficacy and control of hostility and aggressiveness. Gabapentin and pregabalin were well tolerated and effective in controlling anxiety and insomnia, presenting better safety profile and less interactions. Another trial with valproic acid demonstrated efficacy in agitation and aggressiveness but its tolerance was not good and produced a worsening of the cognitive capacity of patients with dementia [34].

We must take special precaution with the use of antipsychotics in nursing home patients, where more than two thirds suffer dementia, and where there is a greater percentage of frail and multi-pathological elderly, leading to more frequent adverse effects and decompensations of the basic pathologies. In a study published by Huybrechts, they compared the risk of serious adverse events among those who continued treatment with an atypical antipsychotic or haloperidol was compared in elderly patients during their stay in residences, using as main variables hospitalization for myocardial infarction, stroke, bacterial infections, or hip fracture [35].

CONCLUSION

The behavioral and psychological symptoms of dementia are a frequent problem, which appears in the different phases of dementia, generating great stress for both the patient and their caregivers.

They constitute a wide group of diverse symptoms, of a psychotic nature: aggressiveness, hallucinations, delusions, erratic wandering; as psychological: apathy, depression, anxiety and insomnia. Therefore, its management must be individualized. Requiring to deepen the clinical history and the patient's exploration, evaluating the impact of these symptoms on the patient and their caregiver.

It should start with non-pharmacological treatment measures, and in this section, an adequate training of caregivers has been shown to reduce the impact of the symptomatology, as well as the recognition of situations that may favor the appearance of them. The activities aimed at physical stimulation, sensory stimulation, psychostimulation or psychorelaxation, and music therapy, keep the patient active with dementia and reduce the appearance of symptoms.

When non-pharmacological measures fail, we must resort to drugs to control the behavioral and psychological symptoms of dementia. There are several therapeutic groups that can be used for this. The most used are antipsychotics. Within this group, haloperidol is the oldest, cheapest and most experienced, and may be useful in the short term. If the symptomatology is maintained or haloperidol is not effective, atypical antipsychotics can be resorted to. Risperidone has shown efficacy in this regard. Other drugs used are anxiolytics if anxiety predominates, or antidepressants, if sadness and depression predominate.

More studies should be conducted to evaluate the efficacy of non-pharmacological measures for the management of these symptoms.

CONSENT FOR PUBLICATION

Not applicable.

ACKNOWLEDGEMENTS

Declare none.

CONFLICT OF INTEREST

The author confirms that this chapter contents have no conflict of interest.

REFERENCES

[1]   Finkel SI, Costa e Silva J, Cohen G, Miller S, Sartorius N. Behavioral and psychological signs and symptoms of dementia: a consensus statement on current knowledge and implications for research and treatment. Int Psychogeriatr 1996; 8 (Suppl. 3): 497-500.
        [http://dx.doi.org/10.1017/S1041610297003943] [PMID: 9154615]

[2]   Lyketsos CG, Carrillo MC, Ryan JM, *et al.* Neuropsychiatric symptoms in Alzheimer's disease. Alzheimers Dement 2011; 7(5): 532-9.
        [http://dx.doi.org/10.1016/j.jalz.2011.05.2410] [PMID: 21889116]

[3]   Olazaran-Rodriguez J, Agüera-Ortiz LF, Muñiz-Schwochert R. Sintomas psicologicos y conductuales de la demencia: prevencion, diagnostico y tratamiento. Rev Neurol 2012; 55(10): 598-608.
        [PMID: 23143961]

[4]   Kales HC, Gitlin LN, Lyketsos CG. Assessment and management of behavioral and psychological symptoms of dementia. BMJ 2015; 350: h369.
        [http://dx.doi.org/10.1136/bmj.h369] [PMID: 25731881]

[5]   Cummings JL, Mega M, Gray K, Rosenberg-Thompson S, Carusi DA, Gornbein J. The Neuropsychiatric Inventory: comprehensive assessment of psychopathology in dementia. Neurology 1994; 44(12): 2308-14.
        [http://dx.doi.org/10.1212/WNL.44.12.2308] [PMID: 7991117]

[6]   Vilalta Frande J, Lozano Gallego M, Hernández Ferrándiz M, Llinás Reglá J, López Pousa S, López OL, *et al.* NPI propiedades psicométricas de su adaptación al español. Rev Esp Neurol 1995; 29(1): 15-9.

[7]   Lyketsos C. Neuropaychiatric symptoms behavioral and psychological symptoms of dementia and the development of dementia treatments. Intern Psychogeriatrics 2007; 19(3): 409-20.

[8]   Petrovic M, Hurt C, Collins D, *et al.* Clustering of behavioural and psychological symptoms in dementia (BPSD): a European Alzheimer's disease consortium (EADC) study. Acta Clin Belg 2007; 62(6): 426-32.
        [http://dx.doi.org/10.1179/acb.2007.062] [PMID: 18351187]

[9]   Cooper C, Balamurali T, Selwood A, Livingston G. A systematic review of intervention studies about anxiety in caregivers of people with dementia. Int J Geriatr Psychiatry 2006; 48: 477-84.
        [PMID: 17006872]

[10]   Matilla-Mora R, Martínez-Piédrola RM, Fernández Huete J. Eficacia de la terapia ocupacional y otras terapias no farmacológicas en el deterioro cognitivo y la enfermedad de Alzheimer. Rev Esp Geriatr Gerontol 2016; 51(6): 349-56.
        [http://dx.doi.org/10.1016/j.regg.2015.10.006] [PMID: 26613656]

[11]   Abraha I, Rimland JM, Trotta FM, *et al.* Systematic review of systematic reviews of non-pharmacological interventions to treat behavioural disturbances in older patients with dementia. The

SENATOR-OnTop series. BMJ Open 2017; 7(3): e012759.
[http://dx.doi.org/10.1136/bmjopen-2016-012759] [PMID: 28302633]

[12] Jiménez-Palomares M, Rodríguez-Mansilla J, González-López-Arza MV, Rodríguez-Domínguez MT, Prieto-Tato M. Beneficios de la musicoterapia como tratamiento no farmacológico y de rehabilitación en la demencia moderada. Rev Esp Geriatr Gerontol 2013; 48(5): 238-42.
[http://dx.doi.org/10.1016/j.regg.2013.01.008] [PMID: 24053988]

[13] Thomas KS, Baier R, Kosar C, Ogarek J, Trepman A, Mor V. Individaulized music program is associated with improved outcomes for US Nursing Home Residents with dementia 2017.

[14] Cabrera E, Sutcliffe C, Verbeek H, *et al.* On behalf of RightTimePlaceCare consortium "Non-pharmacological interventios as a best practice strategy in people with demenctia living in nursing homes. A systematics review". Eur Geriatr Med 2015; 6: 134-50.
[http://dx.doi.org/10.1016/j.eurger.2014.06.003]

[15] Hsu TJ, Tsai HT, Hwang AC, Chen LY, Chen LK. Predictors of non-pharmacological intervention effect on cognitive function and behavioral and psychological symptoms of older people with dementia. Geriatr Gerontol Int 2017; 17 (Suppl. 1): 28-35.
[http://dx.doi.org/10.1111/ggi.13037] [PMID: 28436192]

[16] Cammisuli DM, Danti S, Bosinelli F, Cipriani G. Non-pharmacological interventios for people with Alzheimers's disease: A critical review of the scientific literaure form de last ten years. Eur Geriatr Med 2016; 7: 57-64.
[http://dx.doi.org/10.1016/j.eurger.2016.01.002]

[17] Walderman G, Gauthier S, Jones R, Wilkinson D, Cummings J, Lopez O. Effecto fo donepezil on emergence of apathy in mild to moderata Alzheimer's disease. Int J Geriatr Psychiatry 2011; 23: 150-7.

[18] Figiel G, Sadowsky C. A systematic review of the effectiveness of rivastigmine for the treatment of behavioral disturbances in dementia and other neurological disorders. Curr Med Res Opin 2008; 24(1): 157-66.
[http://dx.doi.org/10.1185/030079908X260961] [PMID: 18036286]

[19] Tangwongchai S, Thavichachart N, Senanarong V, *et al.* Galantamine for the treatment of BPSD in Thai patients with possible Alzheimer's disease with or without cerebrovascular disease. Am J Alzheimers Dis Other Demen 2008; 23(6): 593-601.
[http://dx.doi.org/10.1177/1533317508320603] [PMID: 18845693]

[20] Grossberg GT, Pejović V, Miller ML, Graham SM. Memantine therapy of behavioral symptoms in community-dwelling patients with moderate to severe Alzheimer's disease. Dement Geriatr Cogn Disord 2009; 27(2): 164-72.
[http://dx.doi.org/10.1159/000200013] [PMID: 19194105]

[21] Visado del Ministerio de Sanidad español para el uso de antipsicóticos atípicos publicacionessangvaes/cas/prof/dgf//II_2005-12_enero_antipsicoticosatipicospd

[22] Agüera Ortiz L, Moríñigo Domínguez A, Olivera Pueyo J, Pla Vidal J, Azanda JR. Documento de la SEPG sobre el uso de antipsicóticos en personas de edad avanzada. Psicogeriatría 2017; 7 (Suppl. 1): S1-S37.

[23] Hereu P, Vallano A. Uso de antipsicóticos en pacientes con demencia. Rev Esp Geriatr Gerontol 2011; 46(1): 50-3.
[http://dx.doi.org/10.1016/j.regg.2010.11.003] [PMID: 21315489]

[24] Lonergan E, Luxenberg J, Coldford J, Birks J. Haloperidol para la agitación en la demencia". Cochrane Database os. Syst Rev 2002; (2): CD002852.

[25] Kales HC, Kim HM, Zivin K, *et al.* Risk of mortality among individual antipsychotics in patients with dementia. Am J Psychiatry 2012; 169(1): 71-9.
[http://dx.doi.org/10.1176/appi.ajp.2011.11030347] [PMID: 22193526]

[26]   Ballard CG, Waite G, Birks J. Atypical antipsychotics for aggression and psychosis in Alzheimer's disease. Cochrane Database Syst Rev 2006; (1): CD003476.
       [PMID: 16437455]

[27]   Schneider L, Dagerman K, Insel P. Efficacy and adverse effects of atypical antipsychotic s for dementia: Meta-analysis of randomized, placebo controlled trials. Am J Geriatr Psychiatry 2006; 123.

[28]   Schneider L, Tariot P, Dagerman K, *et al.* Effectiveness of atypical antipsychotic drugs in patients with Alzheimer's disease 2006.

[29]   Durán JC, Greenspan A, Diago JI, Gallego R, Martinez G. Evaluation of risperidone in the treatment of behavioral and psychological symptoms and sleep disturbances associated with dementia. Int Psychogeriatr 2005; 17(4): 591-604.
       [http://dx.doi.org/10.1017/S104161020500219X] [PMID: 16202185]

[30]   Baskys A. Lewy body dementia: the litmus test for neuroleptic sensitivity and extrapyramidal symtoms

[31]   Byrne EJ, O'Brien J. "The treatment of dementia with Lewy bodies". Ames D, Burns A, O'Brien J Dementia 4th ed. 2010; 620-8.

[32]   Porsteinsson AP, Drye LT, Pollock BG, *et al.* Effect of citalopram on agitation in Alzheimer disease: the CitAD randomized clinical trial. JAMA 2014; 311(7): 682-91.
       [http://dx.doi.org/10.1001/jama.2014.93] [PMID: 24549548]

[33]   Lopez Pousa S, García Olmo J. Vilalta Franch, Turon _Estrada a, Pericot I. "Trazodone for Alzheimer's disease: a naturalistic follow-up study. Arch Gerontol Geriatr 2007.

[34]   Olin JT, Fox LS, Pawluczyk S, Taggart NA, Schneider LS. A pilot randomized trial of carbamazepine for behavioral symptoms in treatment-resistant outpatients with Alzheimer disease. Am J Geriatr Psychiatry 2001; 9(4): 400-5.
       [http://dx.doi.org/10.1097/00019442-200111000-00008] [PMID: 11739066]

[35]   Huybrechts KF, Schneeweiss S, Gerhard T, *et al.* Comparative safety of antipsychotic medications in nursing home residents. J Am Geriatr Soc 2012; 60(3): 420-9.
       [http://dx.doi.org/10.1111/j.1532-5415.2011.03853.x] [PMID: 22329464]

CHAPTER 10

Action of Nurses to Improve Prospective Memory in People Affected by Alzheimer's

Borja González-Morales[1], María del Mar Ponferrada Vivanco[1], María del Carmen Ruiz-González[2] and Jacinto Escobar Navas[3,*]

[1] *Resident Nurse of Mental Health, Hospital Universitario Virgen de las Nieves, Granada, Spain*

[2] *Resident Nurse of Mental Health, Health & Sciences Technology Park Hospital Granada, Spain*

[3] *President of the Official College of Nursing of Granada, Granada, Spain*

Abstract: In Alzheimer's disease, the person may suffer a significant cognitive impairment, and one of the most common problems within them is memory loss, which may be seriously compromised. Usually, retrograde amnesia occurs at an advanced stage of the disease. However, anterograde amnesia usually occurs in early episodes of the process, and must have strategies to decrease its progression. People affected by Alzheimer's, due to the characteristics of the pathology, will need continued care in the course of the disease and, moreover, the nurses should have training in this area to help patients improve their prospective memory. In an exhaustive review of the literature, there are interventions that the nurses can do independently with the patient, and other interventions that can do in an interdisciplinary way, along with other professionals.

Keywords: Anterograde Amnesia, Alzheimer's Disease, Memory, Nursing Research.

NURSING CARE IN ALZHEIMER'S DISEASE

German psychiatrist Alois Alzheimer, at the beginning of the 20th century, defined what a century later would become known as the "silent epidemic of the 21st century". Alzheimer's disease (AD) is a neurodegenerative organic pathology of cortical origin, with progressive and insidious onset, defined by memory loss, limitation in the resolution of problems and difficulty in understanding, as well as certain behavioral alterations. Certainly, it is a serious public health problem as in 2015, according to Spanish Statistical Office (INE), is the fifth leading cause of morbidity and mortality in Spain and one of the diseases with the most impact at the family level. The onset of AD in a relative requires the restructuring of the

* **Corresponding author Jacinto Escobar Navas:** Official College of Nursing of Granada, Granada, Spain; Tel: +34 958275700; E-mail: jacinto.escobar@sjd.es

family system changing roles, assuming losses and facing various negative feelings such as depression and anxiety [1].

Therefore, the presence of a good socio-sanitary team, in particular, nurses, is important. The needs that arise in this pathology are palliated with long-term care. These cares will be aimed at providing welfare to the patient and his family, taking care to add quality to life, taking care to prevent the suffering and pain, and taking care to live and die with dignity.

Nutritional needs in a patient with AD may be very compromised by problems when ingesting, chewing or swallowing in addition to the great loss of appetite. It will be necessary to support self-care in feeding, partial or total, securing a postural hygiene in food and maintain a suitable environment. Precautions must be taken in order to prevent aspiration, monitor swallowing and maintain a semi-soft meal for easy chewing [2].

At the digestive level, it can be associated with periods of constipation and difficult elimination related to low mobility and even a deficit in fluid intake. The support of self-care in the toilet, always respecting privacy, and help the patient by establishing specific intervals to set a routine will be essential. When the incontinence is total, this need will be supplied performing perianal washes with warm water and neutral soap, placing a new absorbent, keeping both the bed and surroundings clean. We must not forget the handling of the impaction and constipation, where fluid intake is important.

As the disease progress, strength and energy will be reduced, there being instability in the motion and low tolerance to activity. In early stages, care will be made through therapies that stimulate the exercise and use assistive devices for ambulate and move, if necessary. Joint movements and massages are important to prevent muscular atrophy and the risk of ulcers [3].

In more advanced stages, care shall be taken to the bedridden patient. Firstly, antithrombotic measures shall be taken to avoid risks and prevent ulcers by pressure through devices such as anti-decubitus mattresses and stimulation, as well as helping the patient, who is already highly dependent, in basic activities as nutrition or hygiene.

For patients with AD, it can be very difficult to fall asleep and even keep sleep, waking up several times in one night. Nursing care should focus on improving restful sleep. We must promote a comfortable environment without light or noise and it is important to take hygiene and nutritional measures like brushing his teeth or not have heavy meals before bedtime. Do not allow the patient sleep during the day to feel tired at night and avoid interruptions. Many times, the use of sedative and hypnotic medication is necessary to avoid psychomotor agitation [3].

At the cognitive level not only memory is affected. Also occurs an alteration of the language and there is an executive dysfunction such as aprosexia (inability to fix the attention), agnosia (limitation or inability to interpret stimuli), visuospatial deficits, and sometimes also can be psychotic symptoms, such as delusions and hallucinations.

Among the interventions most appropriate that nursing can do, we find the therapy orientation to reality, where we will work the three areas: orientation in person, time and space. Cognitive stimulation exercises have also proved effective: reading and writing, exercises where it is necessary to perform calculations, written memory works, *etc.* When the person affected by Alzheimer's does not find the words in the communication, we can help him complete the sentences, but it is not recommended to point out or insist on this deficit, as it can be an important source of frustration [4].

We must not forget the emotional aspect. In the early stages, depressive episodes and generalized apathy often occur when awareness of the loss of functionality maintains a good cognitive state. This results in the appearance of anxiety-depression syndrome, which can lead to attempts of autolysis. We must show an active listening and quiet attitude when the patient is more agitated. Use kinaesthetic communication, that is, through body language, to facilitate the understanding of information, so that the patient focuses the attention on the message we want to convey. With our presence, combining appropriate postures and gestures, we can generate a feeling of tranquillity. For this reason, we will avoid sudden movements that can be understood as a signal of aggressiveness and reduce their concentration. It is important the contact and closeness with the patient, be sympathetic with the situation and making emphatic statements of support and affection. We must increase the coping especially in early stages, show support in his decision making and when not possible, the family must do it. There may be a large family dysfunctions and conflicts that are awakened by taking care of a highly dependent person due to the overload that this entails. So, we must show a lot of support, especially to the primary caregiver doing intermittent care that can ease him the burden [2, 4].

NEED OF SPECIALIZED CARE

Organizations such as the Pan American Health Organization and the World Health Organization speak of the need for training nurses regarding diagnostics and assessments based on the needs of patients diagnosed from Alzheimer's disease. They also highlight that there is evidence of the low proportion of staff receiving training in the care of dementias, even in professionals who work in specialized services in these pathologies [5].

In the Mental Health Strategy of the Spanish Health System 2009-2013 dementias and serious cognitive disorders are considered within the most serious and prevalent mental disorders.

In this same strategy it is mentioned that the professionalization of nursing specialist in mental health is an essential element for the development of services and it is admitted that this is developing slowly, because, although nurses have been trained for years in mental health, only some services offer positions with specialist category. The strategy also recommends that the autonomous communities include the qualification of the specialist in mental health nursing as a requisite for the incorporation to jobs in mental health devices and resources [6].

The second edition of the *Consenso Español sobre Demencias* [Spanish Consensus on Dementias], carried out by the Spanish Society of Psychiatry and the Spanish Psychogeriatric Society, defends that the Primary Care Team and the Mental Health Teams constitute the key instruments in the necessary joint approach to dementia. The Mental Health Team must have a mental health nurse in addition as well as other workers [7].

NURSING INTERVENTIONS TO IMPROVE PROSPECTIVE MEMORY IN PEOPLE AFFECTED BY ALZHEIMER

Although the availability of some treatments used at the palliative level, the curative treatment of Alzheimer's disease is not currently possible. For this reason, nursing interventions are an important resource in the treatment of patients, relatives and caregivers. Unlike other diseases, Alzheimer's disease causes a lack of memory that leaves patients in a state of helplessness and despair, and this can lead to unexpected behaviors. The fact that nurses cannot prevent these behaviors can lead to erroneous interventions, such as excessive use of medication or patient abuse or neglect.

To facilitate cognitive functioning there are some stimulatory therapies such as physical exercise, cognitive training and socialization. Physical exercise improves brain circulation and influences executive function (planning, coordination, working memory, abstract thinking, initiation of the right actions and inhibition of inappropriate actions), which requires a lot of brain intervention and has a great deterioration in Alzheimer's disease [2].

The nurses have a series of interventions called Nursing Interventions Classification (NIC), which includes the activities that a nurse is qualified to do and are represented by numerical codes. The most appropriate nursing interventions to work memory in people suffering from Alzheimer's are the following:

• 4760 Memory Training (to improve memory).

• 4720 Cognitive Stimulation (to promote awareness and understanding of the environment through the use of planned stimuli).

• 4820 Reality Orientation (promotion of the patient's awareness of personal identity, time and environment).

• 4860 Reminiscence Therapy (use of memory of past events, feelings and thoughts in order to facilitate pleasure, quality of life or adaptation to current circumstances).

• 5520 Learning Facilitation (promotion of capacity to process and understand information) [8].

INTERDISCIPLINARY INTERVENTIONS TO IMPROVE PROSPECTIVE MEMORY IN PEOPLE AFFECTED BY ALZHEIMER'S

As we have seen, episodic memory in people suffering from Alzheimer's may be severely affected and retrograde and anterograde amnesia may occur.

Retrograde amnesia is one in which facts and events of the past are not remembered prior to the time of injury or beginning of the disorder, while anterograde amnesia is one in which the information is not stored in the long-term memory after the moment of the injury and this information decays and is forgotten minutes or seconds later.

It is, in addition, one of the first symptoms indicative of the suffering of this dementia: first of all, anterograde amnesia takes place, and later in a more advanced stage of deterioration, retrograde amnesia may occur.

In relation to the first, that is, with the difficulty of remembering new information, there is the so-called prospective memory, which refers to the ability to carry out a future action without an express order to remember it. This type of memory is also affected in patients with Alzheimer's [9].

However, in the scientific literature there are numerous studies focused on retrospective memory, which show that it is less deteriorated than prospective one because the self-initiated mental activities, although difficult to achieve with this pathology, are compensated with environmental keys, something that happens in reverse in the prospective memory (high difficulty to initiate a mental activity and low environmental support).

Therefore, the need to specifically investigate the problems of prospective memory in people affected by Alzheimer's is evident, since it is essential for individuals to reach reasonable functionality and be able to live successfully in the community, thus substantially increasing their quality of life [10 - 12].

This review of current scientific evidence focuses primarily on strategies and activities that nurses can perform to improve prospective memory in patients with Alzheimer's. Prospective memory failures may occur in the intention formation stage (*i. e.*, the coding phase), the period of delay between the formation of the intention and the detection of the memory signal (*i. e.*, the storage phase) and signal detection and automatically initiated recovery stage (*i. e.*, recovery phase). While we recognize that there is a considerable theoretical debate about the independence of these "stages", they provide a useful heuristic model around which to organize a discussion of possible treatment and improvement approaches [13].

CODING

One of the most effective interventions that are included in the bibliography is the implementation of intentions formulated by Gollwitzer. It is based on defining a situation in advance with certain actions that we will carry out in this case, so that a situation / action association occurs, and the cognitive effort is reduced to carry it out: "if X occurs, I will do Y" [13]. It has been shown that the implementation of intentions is effective to increase the likelihood that people will have regular blood glucose tests, take vitamin C pills and automate certain processes that require a mild-moderate cognitive demand [14].

Another method with greater relevance is spaced recovery method. This technique consists in recovering the information gradually through longer and longer delay intervals. Its effectiveness has been attributed to priming, operant conditioning, classical conditioning and learning without errors, but there is a general consensus that most of its improvement effects are due to automatic processing. In a study involving a group of healthy adults and another group with cognitive impairment who underwent tests of spaced recovery, adults with cognitive impairment showed a more remarkable improvement in prospective memory than healthy adults [15].

Another study in the same line, investigated in two groups of adults -some healthy and others with Alzheimer's- the effectiveness of the recovery spaced by itself or combined with the elaborated coding of the task. It was shown that 63% of the participants with Alzheimer's performed the combined task better than the spaced recovery alone, so it would be appropriate to use it in combination with other methods [16].

In an investigation carried out by Pereira *et al.*, it was proposed to study the prospective memory enhancement through physical representation when coding the activities. They demonstrated that motor activity during coding improved the likelihood of recall of such activity, rather than if the coding was merely verbal in a statistically significant way. Even semantic coding is also related to a higher probability of recall [17].

STORAGE

With regard to storage, the most outstanding technique is training in the management of objectives, formulated by Levine *et al.* It is an innovative method in the sense that it uses structured group exercises, not relegating to the individual, in which the executive difficulties that each one of the members of the group have and the common experiences are highlighted in order to discover strategies among all of them which can improve recall, such as using mental images, pausing to stop and think, writing to-do lists, recording successes and errors, recording factors related to better or worse performance (distractions, time pressure, realistic planning, low mood) [18]. It has been shown that this method is much more effective if it is combined with the detention technique, which involves linking the keyword "STOP" with a break in the activity that takes place at a given time, reviewing the objectives that were raised prior to the realization of such activity. This keyword is presented by electronic alarms (for example, text messages or reminders of a mobile phone), so that they serve as environmental support to think about the objectives that were previously formulated [13].

RECOVERY

The use of new technologies is promoting a breakthrough in this field. In the same line, a study carried out with a patient used Google Calendar to create alarms. It was shown that this tool produces a significant improvement of the prospective memory by acting as an external alarm, however, it requires technology knowledge and management prior to its use [19].

In the literature there are also newer methods, such as the game of the virtual week. This game consists in simulating tasks of daily life during a week (for example, remember to take the medication), some are performed more regularly and others with less frequency [20]. A study of twelve sessions of one hour each was carried out during a month, in which the game of the virtual week was applied with an experimental group and a control group with which the virtual week task was not carried out. It was shown that the experimental group improved significantly in the short term with respect to the control group, in measures of prospective memory, so that the simulation of daily tasks through the game of the virtual week is postulated as an effective intervention to work the prospective memory in patients with Alzheimer's [20, 21]. There are other investigations that not only focus on prospective memory, but also include working memory. It is the so-called breakfast task, formulated by Craik and Bialystok, who concluded that this task was an indicator of the overall planning of the user, and in turn were related to individual differences in working memory performance and prospective memory. It consists of a computer program, in which the preparation of a breakfast is simulated, cooking five foods that were not well done nor rare, but were ready to serve. The participants had to press a "start" button when they started the task and "stop" buttons that were located right next to the food where the cooking state of the food appeared with a timer in real time. Between the starting and stopping of the cooking, the user had to perform a distracting task, which in this case was to set the table. In the study by Rose *et al.*, it is shown that the task of breakfast is effective in evaluating and improving working memory, prospective memory and planning capacity not only in the laboratory, but also as an ecologically valid task and it is also nice to perform [22]. Finally, other methods that have been proven effective in the literature are the verbal reminders from other people and direct observation therapy, based on family or health professionals exercising an environmental key to stimulate the prospective memory of the person affected by Alzheimer's. However, this approach requires significant human resources that are not easily accessible [13].

CONCLUSIONS

In Alzheimer's disease, prospective memory can be severely affected from the early stages of the disease. This occurs because normally there is a marked difficulty in initiating mental activities, which is accompanied by low environmental support that leads to a greater difficulty in carrying out actions in the future. Failures in prospective memory can occur in any of the 3 stages of memory: coding, storage or recovery.

In terms of coding, the most effective interventions have proven to be the implementation of intentions (association between situation and action), the spaced recovery (retrieving information in ever longer intervals, especially, if combined with the elaborated coding of the task) and the simultaneous execution of motor activity during coding.

Regarding storage, it is remarkable the training in the management of objectives, which is a technique that is done at the group level, where the members launch their proposals as a brainstorming of the strategies that help them most (mental images, writing to-do lists, recording successes and errors), especially when used with the detention technique, which consists in associating the word "STOP" when a specific activity is carried out to review the objectives that were proposed at its beginning and that is remembered through environmental support, such as memories through technological devices.

In the third place, measures related to recovery are proposed, such as Google Calendar alarms (remembering through notification), virtual games, the Breakfast Task (where cognitive stimulation is performed) and direct observation therapy. Other people, such as family members.

Finally, it should be noted that the nurse can work certain NICs independently, such as Memory Training, Cognitive Stimulation, Reality Orientation, Reminiscence Therapy and Learning Facilitation, among others.

CONSENT FOR PUBLICATION

Not applicable.

CONFLICT OF INTEREST

The authors declare no conflict of interest, financial or otherwise.

ACKNOWLEDGEMENTS

Declared none.

REFERENCES

[1]   Sagués A, García JM, Suárez R, *et al.* Andalusian Plan of Alzheimer 2007-2010. Health department. Regional government of Andalusia 2007.

[2]   Garcia S, Garcia MJ, Illán CR, *et al.* Intervenciones enfermeras dirigidas a los pacientes de Alzheimer y a sus cuidadores una revisión bibliográfica. Revista Enfermería Docente 2013; 101: 36-40.

[3]   Cuidados continuados en atención primaria a personas con enfermedad de Alzheimer. 1st ed., Madrid: PWC 2013.

[4]   Balvas MV. El profesional de enfermería y el Alzheimer. Revista Nure Investigación 2005; 13: 4-7.

[5]   Dementia: a public health priority. Washington, DC: PAHO 2013.

[6]   Social Policy and Equality Mental Health Strategy of the Spanish Health System 2009-2013. Madrid: Spanish Ministry of Health, Social Policy and Equality 2011.

[7]   Consenso Español sobre Demencias. 2nd ed., Barcelona: Exter 2005.

[8]   Bulechek G, Butcher H, Dochterman J, Wagner C. Nursing interventions classification (NIC). 6th ed., St. Louis: Elsevier 2013.

[9]   El Haj M, Antoine P, Nandrino JL, Kapogiannis D. Autobiographical memory decline in Alzheimer's disease, a theoretical and clinical overview. Ageing Res Rev 2015; 23(Pt B): 183-92.
      [http://dx.doi.org/10.1016/j.arr.2015.07.001] [PMID: 26169474]

[10]   Henry JD, MacLeod MS, Phillips LH, Crawford JR. A meta-analytic review of prospective memory and aging. Psychol Aging 2004; 19(1): 27-39.
[http://dx.doi.org/10.1037/0882-7974.19.1.27] [PMID: 15065929]

[11]   Thompson CL, Henry JD, Withall A, Rendell PG, Brodaty H. A naturalistic study of prospective memory function in MCI and dementia. Br J Clin Psychol 2011; 50(4): 425-34.
[http://dx.doi.org/10.1111/j.2044-8260.2010.02004.x] [PMID: 22003951]

[12]   Woods SP, Weinborn M, Li YR, Hodgson E, Ng AR, Bucks RS. Does prospective memory influence quality of life in community-dwelling older adults? Neuropsychol Dev Cogn B Aging Neuropsychol Cogn 2015; 22(6): 679-92.
[http://dx.doi.org/10.1080/13825585.2015.1027651] [PMID: 25808599]

[13]   Zogg JB, Woods SP, Sauceda JA, Wiebe JS, Simoni JM. The role of prospective memory in medication adherence: a review of an emerging literature. J Behav Med 2012; 35(1): 47-62.
[http://dx.doi.org/10.1007/s10865-011-9341-9] [PMID: 21487722]

[14]   Chasteen AL, Park DC, Schwarz N. Implementation intentions and facilitation of prospective memory. Psychol Sci 2001; 12(6): 457-61.
[http://dx.doi.org/10.1111/1467-9280.00385] [PMID: 11760131]

[15]   Ozgis S, Rendell PG, Henry JD. Spaced retrieval significantly improves prospective memory performance of cognitively impaired older adults. Gerontology 2009; 55(2): 229-32.
[http://dx.doi.org/10.1159/000163446] [PMID: 18843179]

[16]   Kinsella GJ, Ong B, Storey E, Wallace J, Hester R. Elaborated spaced-retrieval and prospective memory in mild Alzheimer's disease. Neuropsychol Rehabil 2007; 17(6): 688-706.
[http://dx.doi.org/10.1080/09602010600892824] [PMID: 17852763]

[17]   Pereira A, de Mendonça A, Silva D, Guerreiro M, Freeman J, Ellis J. Enhancing prospective memory in mild cognitive impairment: The role of enactment. J Clin Exp Neuropsychol 2015; 37(8): 863-77.
[http://dx.doi.org/10.1080/13803395.2015.1072499] [PMID: 26313515]

[18]   Fish J, Wilson BA, Manly T. The assessment and rehabilitation of prospective memory problems in people with neurological disorders: a review. Neuropsychol Rehabil 2010; 20(2): 161-79.
[http://dx.doi.org/10.1080/09602010903126029] [PMID: 20146135]

[19]   El Haj M, Gallouj K, Antoine P. Google calendar enhances prospective memory in Alzheimer's Disease: A case report. J Alzheimers Dis 2017; 57(1): 285-91.
[http://dx.doi.org/10.3233/JAD-161283] [PMID: 28222535]

[20]   Rose NS, Rendell PG, McDaniel MA, Aberle I, Kliegel M. Age and individual differences in prospective memory during a "Virtual Week": the roles of working memory, vigilance, task regularity, and cue focality. Psychol Aging 2010; 25(3): 595-605.
[http://dx.doi.org/10.1037/a0019771] [PMID: 20853967]

[21]   Rose NS, Rendell PG, Hering A, Kliegel M, Bidelman GM, Craik FI. Cognitive and neural plasticity in older adults' prospective memory following training with the Virtual Week computer game. Front Hum Neurosci 2015; 9(592): 1-13.
[PMID: 26578936]

[22]   Rose NS, Luo L, Bialystok E, Hering A, Lau K, Craik FI. Cognitive processes in the Breakfast Task: Planning and monitoring. Can J Exp Psychol 2015; 69(3): 252-63.
[http://dx.doi.org/10.1037/cep0000054] [PMID: 25938251]

SUBJECT INDEX

Computed tomography (CT) 17, 73, 83, 84
Confidence interval 26, 27, 109, 125, 128
Consciousness 110, 111, 113, 115, 116
  level of 113, 115, 116
Consent, explicit 111
Constipation 37, 41, 148, 153, 164
Coronal plane 83, 84, 87
Coronary 5, 125
  disease 5
  heart disease 125
Cortex, cerebral 17, 90, 92
Cortical atrophy, global 84, 86
Creutzfeldt-Jakob disease (CJD) 71, 73

D

Dairy products 124, 125, 134
Data sheet, technical 114, 115
DCL and atypical dementia 92
Decision making 98, 104, 165
  in advanced dementia 104
Default mode network (DMN) 19, 20, 23
Degenerative 68, 83, 144, 154
  dementia type 154
  diseases 68, 83, 144
  neurological 83
Deglutition disorders 98
Delusions 36, 144, 145, 147, 154, 159, 165
Dementia 21, 23, 43, 53, 92, 98, 106, 107, 108,
    110, 135, 151, 153, 154
  cortical 53
  developing 21, 135
  diagnosed 1
  institutionalized 153
  late-stage 108
  moderate-severe 154
  progressive degenerative 92
  severe 23, 43, 53, 106, 107, 108, 110, 151
  terminal 98
Dementia patients 36, 38, 52, 101, 135, 150
  frontotemporal 38
  institutionalized 52
Deposits, amyloid 18, 27, 94, 95

Depression 2, 36, 41, 123, 135, 144, 145, 146, 147,
    155, 158, 159, 164
Deterioration 17, 86, 166, 167
DFT and mild cognitive dementia 73
Diagnosis 69, 83, 123, 128
  differential 69, 83
  etiological 123, 128
Dialysis 109, 110
Diets 62, 63, 130, 131, 132
  crushed 62, 63
  customary 131, 132
  low-fat 130
Diffusion imaging (DTI) 20, 24, 28, 92
Disease 20, 35, 52, 55, 60, 64, 67, 69, 76, 88, 130,
    133, 144, 146, 149, 158, 164
  cardiovascular 130
  cerebrovascular 67, 76, 88, 133
  dementias 146
  endocrine 144
  infectious 149
  neuro-degenerative 60
  neurologic 52
  neurological 60
  neuromuscular 55
  vasculocerebral 158
Disorders, cognitive 129, 166
Distressing symptoms, common 99, 107
Donepezil 75, 154
Down's syndrome (DS) 4
Drugs 98, 107, 110, 111
  anti-dementia 98, 107
  deliberate administration of 110, 111
Dysphagia 52, 53, 54, 55, 56, 57, 58, 60, 62, 100, 105
  oropharyngeal 52, 54, 56, 57, 60
  prevalence of 52
Dyspnoea 99, 100, 110, 149

E

Early-onset FAD 3, 4
Efficacy, demonstrated 156, 158
Episode, febrile 99
Esophageal sphincter, upper 57, 58
European Association for Palliative Care (EAPC) 110

Respirations 44
Resting state 19, 21, 22, 23
  network (RSNs) 19
Retrograde amnesia 163, 167
Rey auditory verbal learning test (RAVLT) 130
Risk factors, vascular 130, 131
Risperidone 154, 156, 157, 159

S

Scales 39, 101
  dementia severity 101
  simple 39
Sedation 110, 111, 112, 113, 114, 115, 116, 156
  decision 113, 116
  terminal 114
Sementia 34
Semi-quantitative food frequency questionnaire 125
Senile plaques (SP) 3, 4
Signs, videofluoroscopic 57, 58
Single photon emission computed tomography (SPECT) 83, 91, 94
Solanezumab 7, 74
SPECT in dementia of Alzheimer type 94
Stages 27, 28, 39
  intermediate 39
  prodromal-AD 27, 28
Stimulation, cognitive 153, 167, 171
Stimuli, intense painful 37
Strategies 60, 61, 99
  postural 60, 61
  for care of advanced dementia 99
Stress, oxidative 2, 3, 134
Stroke-Alzheimer's disease 128
Structural connectivity (SC) 20
Subcomponents 20
Subcutaneous route 98, 114, 115, 116
Subjective cognitive decline (SCD) 17, 18, 23, 24
Suffering advanced dementia 103
Supplements, high-calorie 105
Support system 103

Surrogates 63, 64
Swallowing, safety and efficacy of 56, 57
Symptomatology 2, 146, 153, 159
Symptoms 1, 69, 111, 114, 147, 153, 157, 158, 165
  cognitive 1, 69
  depressive 147, 153, 158
  psychotic 155, 157, 158, 165
  refractory 111, 114
Syndromes, geriatric 35, 53
System, lateral pain 37

T

Task, cognitive 19, 90
Tau aggregation inhibitor (TAI) 9, 10
Tau pathology 8, 9
Tau protein 1, 9, 67, 69, 72, 73, 74, 76
Team, medical 112, 113
Techniques 74, 76, 91, 169, 171
  detention 169, 171
  neuroimaging 74, 76
  perfusion 91
Temporal lobe 83, 85, 88, 90, 93
Tertile, top 129, 133
Tests 17, 18, 54, 92, 126, 128, 131, 132
  included 132
  neuropsychological 17, 18, 92, 126, 128, 131
  screening 54
Therapeutic 1, 3, 4, 5, 9, 108, 109
  procedures, extraordinary 108, 109
  target 1, 3, 4, 5, 9
Therapies 2, 5, 10, 103, 148, 151, 152, 164, 170, 171
  anti-Alzheimer's disease 5
  direct observation 170, 171
  occupational 148, 151, 152
Tolerability profiles 122, 136, 137
Tolerance 37, 38, 157, 158
Tomography, computed 17, 73, 83
Tongue 57, 61
Treatment 1, 2, 43, 60, 136, 144, 148, 150, 153
  non-pharmacological 148, 150, 153
  pharmacological 43, 136, 144, 153
  strategies 2, 60
  symptomatic 1

www.ingramcontent.com/pod-product-compliance
Lightning Source LLC
Chambersburg PA
CBHW041703210326
41598CB00007B/519